THE
SKINNY GUT
DIET

ALSO BY BRENDA WATSON

The Road to Perfect Health

Heart of Perfect Health

The Fiber35 Diet

Gut Solutions

The Detox Strategy

The H.O.P.E. Formula

THE SKINNY GUT DIET

Balance
Your Digestive
System
for Permanent
Weight Loss

BRENDA WATSON,
C.N.C.,
with Jamey Jones, B.Sc., and
Leonard Smith, M.D.

HARMONY
BOOKS · NEW YORK

Copyright © 2014 by Brenda Watson

Published in the United States by Harmony Books, an imprint of the
Crown Publishing Group, a division of Random House LLC,
a Penguin Random House Company, New York.

www.crownpublishing.com

Harmony Books is a registered trademark, and the Circle colophon is a
trademark of Random House LLC.

Library of Congress Cataloging-in-Publication Data is available upon request.

ISBN 978-0-553-41794-4
eBook ISBN 978-0-553-41795-1

Printed in the United States of America

Book design by Lauren Dong
Illustrations by Jim Bayne, FrontRanger.com
Jacket design by Michael Nagin

10 9 8 7 6 5 4 3 2 1

First Edition

To Stan, my husband,
who stands beside me in all ways.

CONTENTS

THE GUT FACTOR—WHAT STANDS BETWEEN YOU AND YOUR SKINNY JEANS?

The obesity epidemic currently facing the nation and most of the rest of the world is reaching a critical point. Chronic disease is rampant as a result of the escalating obesity rate, and for the first time in over a century, the newest generation will be the first to have a lower life expectancy than the last. Not only are adults getting fatter and fatter but so are our children. Yet there are more diets and exercise programs available than ever before. So many people are chronically trying to lose weight, and yet the obesity rate climbs. There seems to be a piece missing from the puzzle.

What would you say if I told you that you have an inner weight-loss secret waiting to be revealed? What if you knew that you are only partly responsible for being overweight, and that even if you do everything you can to get healthy and lose your belly, you won't achieve lasting weight loss if you don't address this one factor? What if you knew that, by addressing this factor, not only would you finally lose weight—and keep it off—but you would also experience the side benefits of fewer digestive problems, a stronger immune system, and even a better mood?

You have likely tried a number of diets by now, losing weight each time only to gain it back—and then some. You have reduced the fat, reduced the sugar, reduced the carbohydrates, and certainly reduced the flavor of your meals. You have counted calories, counted inches, counted pounds, and counted on each diet being the last one you'll ever try. You have eaten mindfully, eaten organically, eaten locally, and eaten your way through more diet books than you care to admit.

But I'm willing to bet that you have not taken into account your inner weight-loss secret. If you knew that you had within you one thing that could change your weight-loss fate for good—and that scientific research could prove it—would you be interested? I'm here to tell you that your inner weight-loss secret lies within your digestive tract. I call it the *gut factor*.

Inside your digestive tract are trillions of bacteria that play a crucial role in not only your digestive and immune health but also your overall health—and most notably, your weight. Each of us has a unique balance of bacteria that either protects us and keeps us healthy or leaves us susceptible to disease. That same balance can contribute to either weight gain or to weight loss. When your gut bacteria are out of balance, you gain weight. Conversely, when you balance your gut by eating the right foods (and by *avoiding* the wrong foods), you lose weight, reduce cravings, ditch digestive upsets, boost immunity, reduce inflammation, and feel great.

At the heart of that digestive balance we find good bacteria: the beneficial microbes found in a healthy digestive tract that work in myriad ways to keep you healthy. By eating living foods—those foods that contain good bacteria (also called probiotics) and foods that feed these bacteria in your gut—you will balance your gut and finally be able to achieve the lasting weight loss you have been seeking.

There are two main groups (phyla) of bacteria in the gut:

- Bacteroidetes (pronounced BAC-ter-OY-deh-tees)
- Firmicutes (fir-MIH-cue-tees)

Don't worry—I don't expect you to remember these long names. Instead, let's call them "Fat bacteria" (Firmicutes) and "Be Skinny bacteria" (Bacteroidetes). Your ratio of these two groups determines whether or not you will be more likely to gain weight. The Firmicutes bacteria are better able to extract calories from food and cause you to accumulate more fat than the Bacteroidetes. Simply put, for weight loss you want to increase the Bacteroidetes and decrease the Firmicutes in your gut.

There are also two smaller groups (genera) of bacteria that are beneficial to your overall health:

- *Bifidobacterium*
- *Lactobacillus*

Bifidobacteria are acquired during infancy and by eating certain foods throughout life. They are found in highest amounts in a healthy colon, or large intestine, and they protect us against infection, boost our immune function, help keep us regular, and produce certain vitamins and nutrients. Lactobacilli are obtained during birth and also by eating particular foods. They are found throughout the digestive tract, but are particularly associated with the health of the small intestine. *Lactobacillus* bacteria help our immune and digestive systems function well, and they are also found in the vaginal tract, where they establish bacterial balance by producing lactic acid and hydrogen peroxide to maintain a healthy pH level there. Both Bifidobacteria and Lactobacilli protect us against an overgrowth of pathogenic bacteria in the intestine. In effect, they "crowd out" the bad bacteria in our guts, promoting gut balance.

All of these beneficial bacteria—Bifidobacteria, Lactobacilli, and many bacteria from the Bacteroidetes group—can be increased in your gut by eating foods that feed these bacteria while starving the bad bacteria. The result will be a gut balance that helps you lose weight and stay healthy. I wrote this book to help spread the word about this inner weight-loss secret because I have seen so many people achieve vibrant health and optimal weight by balancing their guts.

I don't want it to be a secret anymore. You see, digestive health is the foundation for total-body health. If you don't address weight gain at its core—at the gut level—then you can't lose weight and expect to keep it off.

Why are weight-loss goals so difficult to achieve? The answer is simple. Current diet programs do not address the underlying contributor to your weight gain: *the gut factor*. Gut imbalance contributes to a wide range of digestive conditions. And, unfortunately, digestive health is often overlooked. Instead of paying attention to digestive disruptions, we tend to cover our symptoms with medications such as acid blockers and antacids, antibiotics, immune suppressors, anti-inflammatories, and laxatives. These medications merely act to silence symptoms that indicate something is not quite right. Silencing your symptoms does not address the *cause* of your symptoms, however. This is a fundamental problem of conventional medicine.

I propose a different model. Instead of covering up your digestive symptoms with medications laden with side effects (many of which actually cause further digestive damage rather than fix the real problem), why not dig deeper? Why not uncover the true foundational digestive imbalances that, when resolved, eliminate the need for such treatments in the first place?

What if, by balancing your gut bacteria with the right foods, supplements, and lifestyle, you might be able to finally drop the weight that has burdened you for so long? Could the answer really lie within you? Could the bacteria you house within your gut have the power to turn your health around for the better? It sure can. And I will show you how.

The Skinny Gut Diet is a lifestyle that will transform your health by giving you the tools to eat well for your gut, so that you can finally lose weight and feel great. You will learn how to eat foods that nourish you and the population of beneficial bacteria within you. You will discover the three simple rules that make eating healthy easy and delicious. A two-week menu planner will guide your meal decisions and give you inspiration to adapt the diet to your own preferences.

Appealing, easy-to-prepare recipes will help you eat for your gut on a regular basis. A simple supplementation guide will help you round out your diet to keep you nourished from the inside out, and a rescue kit will help you navigate in the world with your new eating habits.

By traveling back to the source of your overall health and addressing the imbalances in your gut, you can fundamentally change the downstream effects that have kept you overweight and unhappy for so long. This book will give you the tools you need to finally shed unwanted weight—both of physical pounds and of unhappiness. I will reveal how the digestive system is the true source of health, and I'll help you put into action the simple steps to balance your gut to achieve your ideal weight and feel your best.

Yours in vibrant health,
Brenda Watson

Chapter 1

A REMARKABLE DISCOVERY—GUESS WHO'S COMING TO DINNER?

It is no secret that your digestive tract performs vital functions that allow your body to work optimally. After all, over the course of a lifetime you will eat over 60 tons of food that must be broken down into nutrients that can be absorbed and used by your body, while the rest—what we usually think of as waste—is removed via bowel movements. Digestive function is hardly a new discovery. What is most remarkable about your digestion, however, is at the microscopic level—your gut microbes, mostly composed of the bacteria within your digestive tract.

Living inside you at this very moment is a community of organisms. You house a literal ecosystem inside your digestive tract made up of 100 trillion microorganisms that outnumber—by ten times!—the individual cells that make up your entire body. Numerically speaking, you are only 10 percent human. The other 90 percent is mostly bacteria along with other microbes such as yeasts, viruses, and, yes, even parasites. In fact, it is no longer plausible to consider yourself as one being. You may now think of yourself in the plural—*we* rather than *I*.

> **The vast majority of your gut microbes are bacteria.**
> **The remaining microbes include yeasts, viruses, and parasites.**

Let me say that again: Your gut contains 100 trillion (with a capital "T") gut bacteria. It's hard even to conceive of so many bacteria. We usually only think of such high numbers when we discuss the national debt—and even the $16 trillion national debt is dwarfed by the magnitude of your bacteria community. Your heart will beat an average of 2.5 billion times in a lifetime, and the average male will eat over 75 million calories before he dies, yet these enormous totals pale in comparison to the number of bacteria living in your gut this very moment.

The bacteria in your gut contain over 100 times more DNA than your own human DNA. Your microbial genes work together with your human genes to keep you healthy or, in certain cases, cause disease. The DNA of your bacteria is unique to you, like a fingerprint, and research shows that your bacterial genes may impact your health even more than your own genes will. You can't see them and you usually can't feel them, but your gut bacteria are in control. Considered an organ in their own right,[1] the microorganisms in your digestive tract perform an astonishing array of functions that are only recently being regarded as an integral component of human health. Once considered simply passengers as they traveled through our intestines, it is now known that not only do our microbes rely on us but, perhaps even more so, we rely on them.

Every surface of your body—both the outer cover of the skin and the inner linings that include the digestive tract, urogenital tract, and even the respiratory tract—is covered in microbes. Researchers worldwide are currently hard at work trying to characterize these microbes and determine their relationship to human health. Their discoveries are turning out to be some of the most exciting medical advances of our time. And they've only begun to scratch the surface.

THE SIX REASONS GUT BACTERIA ARE REMARKABLE

Gut bacteria are remarkable for six main reasons. Your gut bacteria can help you:

1. Lose weight.
2. Keep weight off for good.

3. Reduce silent inflammation (the root cause of chronic disease).
4. Improve immune function.
5. Reduce digestive distress and stay regular.
6. Reduce depression and anxiety.

Pretty remarkable, I would say. Did you have any idea your gut bacteria could do so much? The bacteria in your gut are hard at work, day in and day out, keeping you healthy and protecting you against disease.

If you are reading this book, you are likely facing the same struggle with weight that I have faced—endless dieting, endless cheating, and endless fluctuations of not only weight but the moods and other health conditions along with it. It's a vicious cycle of battles and triumphs, ups and downs, successes and failures. I can tell you, it's exhausting. I've been there. I have ridden the same diet roller coaster as you—until I decided to get off the ride.

I went on a search for the real answer to weight loss and good health. What I found would surprise you. Through my research and experience working with others, I found that the only way to truly achieve lasting weight loss was by looking within and balancing the gut—that is, increasing the beneficial bacteria and decreasing the harmful bacteria. Without gut balance, you will only lose superficial weight and you will only achieve superficial health. By balancing your gut—and addressing your health at its true core—you will be able to finally get to the heart of what ails you physically, mentally, and emotionally, as you will see. Truly, your health begins in your gut.

MY ROAD TO THE SKINNY GUT DIET

Over thirty years ago I started on the road to naturally heal myself of many health conditions that began during my childhood. I suffered from chronic fatigue and migraine headaches, and a range of digestive disorders that persisted into adulthood. Plus, I was overweight.

These health conditions really impacted my life. All these conditions, I learned later, were directly related to my gut. I, perhaps like you, was a child of the antibiotic revolution—I was given antibiotics in early childhood for just about everything. If I had a bad cold or sore throat, I took antibiotics. If I had an earache, there were more antibiotics. Stubbed my toe? Just in case, I took antibiotics. You know the routine.

As a result of too many courses of unnecessary antibiotics, the good bacteria in my digestive system were destroyed, which led to my poor health later in life. After being frustrated for many adult years going to doctors who had no answers for my health problems, I took matters into my own hands and began to seek natural solutions. I became my own health advocate. This was in the 1980s, mind you, when natural health was considered strange at best. But it called out to me because of the central theme that the body should be treated as a whole—that each system is connected to the others, and that there are natural means to help bring balance back to the body.

Today, it's exciting for me to witness how science has expanded our knowledge of the digestive system, particularly how our gut bacteria play a central role in our overall health; just a few decades ago, conventional medicine's view of digestion was comparatively primitive. Studies are continually being published that document gut imbalance (largely due to antibiotic overuse) and its correlation not only to digestive and immune health but also to a broad range of negative health conditions, including diabetes, heart disease, arthritis, mood disorders, and, of course, to the obesity epidemic currently plaguing the nation.

At the start of my journey, I did not know that my gut was the core of my health problems. But I made a decision at that time, based on what I had read in natural health books I found in a health food store, to work on my digestive health so that my overall health would improve. That decision turned out to be one of the biggest and best choices I have ever made. Everything changed when I rebuilt my digestive health. It was like a light went on. By dealing with my inner landscape—by balancing my gut—I was able to finally rid myself of my chronic health conditions. Over a period of time I regained control of my health, weight, energy levels, and the inflammation that was at the root of my problems. Even though the information I had available to me at the time was not backed up with the scientific evidence we have today, it worked. The basic principles of returning the digestive system to health through internal cleansing, healing a leaky gut (more about that later), and restoring the balance of good bacteria are what eventually healed me. Today, science is proving that these principles work.

Restoring my health propelled me into my life's work: to help others do the same. I became an expert in nutrition and natural medicine, earning a degree in natural health and founding five natural health clinics. I wrote nine books and produced five public television shows, as well as gave hundreds of lectures and radio interviews, all about the crucial foundational role of digestive health on overall health. The power of gut health to heal the body is the core of my message, and I share it whenever I can.

This journey has brought me to where I am now—writing *The Skinny Gut Diet* so that I can share my message with you. Over the years I have worked with thousands of people struggling with health issues. In most cases being overweight is a central theme of poor health. A few years ago, in an effort to assist family members, I discovered a new way of helping people with their weight that also had an amazing effect on their health issues. By restoring the balance of friendly bacteria, along with adding foods that feed the good bacteria and removing foods that feed the bad bacteria, people were finally able to drop their weight for good—and their health issues resolved. Blood pressure dropped, cholesterol went down, blood sugar normalized, energy increased, and moodiness disappeared. Since then, I've shared the empowering Skinny Gut Diet program with many people, and it has given them new life.

The Skinny Gut Diet program also changed my own life. I have always known the power of probiotics—these good bacteria have been a part of my health program for many years—but by eating living foods and healthy fats every day, eating protein at each meal and snack, and understanding the importance of tracking my sugar intake (including the sugar that comes from carbohydrates), I have finally been able to keep my weight stable and my inflammation down.

The Skinny Gut Diet is the answer for anyone who wants to not only lose weight but also address the underlying cause of chronic disease—silent inflammation, sometimes referred to as chronic inflammation, which we will talk more about later. I am thrilled to share this program with you. Together, we can achieve vibrant health and optimal weight.

THE WEIGHT-LOSS SECRET WITHIN YOU

Somehow we have been led to believe that fluctuations in weight are the result of a simple energy imbalance resulting from eating too much food and exercising too little. This phenomenon is known as the calories-in/calories-out model, and its validity is being seriously questioned by scientists.[2] The United States is the second-most-obese country in the world, only recently surpassed by Mexico; two-thirds of American adults and one-third of American children are overweight or obese. Many of these people are trying earnestly to eat less and move more, yet their weight continues to climb. Why is it that some people can eat all they want and not get fat, while others count every calorie and regularly work out, only to gain five pounds by looking at a piece of chocolate cake?

The calories-in/calories-out model does not account for the gut factor. As I mentioned at the start, the gut is more densely populated by bacteria than any other part of the body. Researchers are rapidly discovering that these bacteria play an integral role in the development of obesity. In short, the gut factor explains the paradox of our previous understanding of the calories-in/calories-out model.

With the Skinny Gut Diet, you implement a lifestyle that *balances* your gut. You eat delicious foods that feed the beneficial bacteria and reduce the harmful bacteria. You will also take supplements that help maintain that balance and support your core health. Thus, by correcting your imbalance, you will reach a new state of wellness that penetrates deep within you to bring about overall wellness.

How does gut bacterial balance help you lose weight? With the right bacteria:

1. You will absorb fewer extra calories from food.
2. You will store less fat.
3. You will have fewer cravings.

Throughout this book I will be exploring the science behind these points and many more benefits of gut balance—as well as how to achieve that balance by eating fermented foods and fiber and by taking the right supplements. Although the weight-loss benefits of gut balance may be the most important feature for you right now, you will learn that gut balance goes far beyond weight loss. When you balance your gut, you reset your health and you build a strong foundation of wellness.

Diet and Gut Balance—Lost Without Each Other

We can trace obesity back to digestive imbalance in a few ways that are changing how scientists and doctors view this pervasive, epidemic condition—and changing their view of what was once thought to be our useless bacterial inhabitants. Also changing is our view of the role of diet. Once thought to be the major determinant of weight gain or weight loss, it is now clear that our gut bacteria are as important as the foods we eat when it comes to how much weight we will gain and how much fat we will accumulate. In fact, some studies have found that when the gut is in balance, poor diet alone is not enough to induce obesity.[3] But before you get excited about the prospect of being able to eat all you want simply by keeping your gut in balance, know that a poor diet itself will eventually lead to gut imbalance, foiling your plan and packing on the pounds. What's important here is that your gut bacteria and diet *work in conjunction*. You must address both in order to truly regain your health and your waistline. *The Skinny Gut Diet* will help show you how.

The Proof Is in the (Low-Sugar) Pudding

While researching and writing this book, I had the pleasure of guiding ten individuals through the Skinny Gut Diet for a period of three months. I didn't want to just provide you with theory and studies and anecdotal reports. I wanted some hard evidence. So I recruited men and women of varying ages and weights, all of whom needed to lose 20 to 75 pounds. Throughout these pages you will hear the inspiring stories of Eva, Polly, Cynthia, Charlie, Danielle, Alexandra, Dave, Sandi, Theresa, and Shirley. I started them on the diet, and I stayed with them for three months. I am happy to report that, as we go to print, six months later, all participants have maintained or continued to lose weight.

At the beginning of the program, everyone was weighed and measured. But that's not all—they also submitted stool samples to test for gut bacterial imbalances. And, boy, did they have imbalances, as you will read in some of their testimonials! Many had the same gut profile as studies have found in obese people: a high ratio of Fat : Be Skinny bacteria (Firmicutes : Bacteroidetes). Some participants began with high amounts of yeast or other microorganisms, too. Many had relatively low amounts of the beneficial bacteria *Lactobacillus* and *Bifidobacterium*. I suspected as much, since these folks all had 20 to 75 pounds to lose, and I knew that gut imbalance is a root cause of weight gain—the theme of this book.

> **"Prior to the Skinny Gut Diet my brain made my daily food choices; now my healthier gut does." —Eva**

The test we used was the Metametrix GI Effects Comprehensive Profile. This stool test uses both culture-based and DNA-based testing to detect the common beneficial microbes, along with potentially pathogenic microbes, including parasites. And of course, the test measured the Fat : Be Skinny bacteria ratio, also called the adiposity index or fat index. (See graph below.) Participants underwent stool testing at the beginning of the study, after six weeks, and again at three months, when the study ended. Although the idea of submitting a stool sample was not everyone's favorite part of the program, it was a relatively easy process and it gave us a great look at what was going on "inside." Stool testing such as this is truly an eye-opening experience. The idea that we have a vast community within us can seem an elusive concept for most people, but when you see the specifics of what is really going on in there, it can be enlightening and motivating. The following images come from a sample test and are two of the markers that I paid closest attention to in the study participants—the adiposity index and the amount of beneficial *Lactobacillus* and *Bifidobacterium*.

The stool test is helpful to determine how out of balance your gut may be, but it is not a necessary part of the diet. If you are overweight, you likely house the wrong gut microbes. Following the Skinny Gut Diet will help you to replenish the right gut microbes, whether or not a test tells you that you are out of balance.

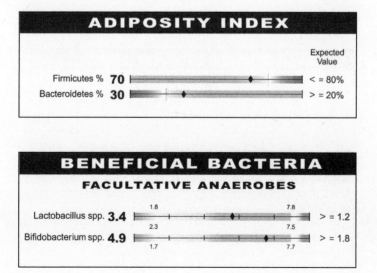

For three months, the Skinny Gut Diet participants followed the three simple rules of the diet:

Rule 1: Eat more fat (healthy fat) to reduce silent inflammation.
Rule 2: Eat living foods every day to balance the gut.

SKINNY GUT SUCCESS STORY: EVA C.

When Eva began the Skinny Gut Diet, she was 52 years old and going through menopause, which doesn't make losing weight any easier. At 5 foot 4 inches and 185 pounds, she found herself 50 pounds away from her ideal weight. Eva is a woman who you would say carries her weight well. But if you asked her, she would tell you she didn't want to carry that weight anymore.

Eva had been challenged with bowel issues for years. Under stress, she would experience loose stool, yet she also dealt with periods of constipation. She regularly felt foggy, with cloudy thinking, bloating, and fatigue.

Eva started out with the characteristic "obese gut type"—high amounts of Firmicutes (Fat bacteria) and lower amounts of Bacteroidetes (Be Skinny bacteria). After just six weeks on the Skinny Gut Diet, her gut resembled the "lean gut type"—her Fat bacteria went down and her Be Skinny bacteria increased.

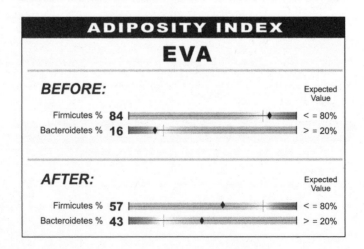

Rule 3: Eat protein at every meal and snack to eliminate cravings.

The participants tracked their daily food intake and did their best to stay within 8 to 10 teaspoons of sugar daily (remember, that

---

"I haven't been in these jeans since 2004! I'm thrilled beyond words." —Eva

On the Skinny Gut Diet, Eva let go of 24 pounds in three months at a gentle and steady pace. Most important, her health improved day by day. Her bowel movements became more regular in frequency and consistency, and she says that her energy, focus, and ability to concentrate are much better. I'm sure you'll agree that those are welcome improvements at any age.

Although the Skinny Gut Diet doesn't address hormonal issues directly, there is no doubt in my mind that a balanced gut supports all functions in the body. The liver is a critical part of the digestive system, and it also performs many hormonal functions. The Skinny Gut Diet removes stress from the liver, allowing it to perform its many other functions more efficiently. I would bet that is why Eva is feeling more clear and energetic, with a sense of overall well-being. I look forward to following Eva's progress through menopause and beyond.

Eva	Weight	Waistline Inches	Body Fat %
Before	189	40½"	43.6%
After	165	36"	39.6%
Lost	24 lbs	4½"	4.0%

number includes the sugar from starchy carbohydrates, too) using the Teaspoon Tracker I developed. This tool was critical in the success of the program and made the diet easy to follow, as participants started to see their food differently. They ate protein at every meal and snack to eliminate cravings. And it worked!

The diet didn't feel restricted. It was simply a new way of eating. The participants learned to eat healthy fats, and they no longer considered *fat* a dirty word. In addition, every day they added the Skinny Gut supplements to their daily routine to optimize digestive health. And it showed. Their digestive symptoms improved and their bowel movements had clockwork regularity. They tracked their weight on a weekly basis, and we measured everyone's waist circumference, waist-to-hip ratio, and percent body fat at the beginning, middle, and end of the study. And down the numbers went, to everyone's delight.

We met almost weekly to check in, share meal ideas and tips, talk about our progress, and touch base as a group on a mission. It was an amazing experience not only for the individuals on the diet but also for me. I never tire of watching people's bodies transform. My opportunity during this time to witness the excitement and engagement of the participants in this program truly brought me joy. The aha! moments came on a regular basis. Indeed, observing the renewal of these individuals was inspiring.

I am writing this book because I want the same renewal for you. I want you to realize that eating healthy and achieving your ideal weight can be simple, once you take into account the gut factor. I hope that you have found inspiration in these pages and that you have already begun the journey back to your true self—the you who is healthy, lean, well-nourished, and most of all, happy.

CHAPTER 1 SUMMARY

Your Inner Ecosystem
- ➤ Your digestive tract contains 100 trillion microorganisms—ten times the number of cells that make up your entire body.
- ➤ Your health is not so much under your control as under the control of your bacteria.

Gut bacteria are remarkable because they help you:
- ➤ Lose weight.
- ➤ Keep weight off for good.
- ➤ Reduce depression and anxiety.
- ➤ Reduce digestive distress and stay regular.
- ➤ Reduce silent inflammation (the root cause of chronic disease).
- ➤ Balance immune function.

The Skinny Gut Diet helps you balance your gut so that you will:
- ➤ Absorb fewer extra calories from food.
- ➤ Store less fat.
- ➤ Have fewer cravings.

Chapter 2

GUT BACTERIA—THE SURPRISING WEIGHT-LOSS SOLUTION

M y sister Sandee has always worked really hard to stay healthy. She is in her fifties and, like most of us baby boomers, she gradually put on weight over the years. Fortunately, Sandee was already aware of the benefits of taking probiotics, but she wasn't helping to maintain that balance with her diet. You see, Sandee had a sugar addiction.

> Gut microbes help give a new twist to the phrase "You are what you eat." You are what your gut microbes do with what you eat.

Sandee started her morning with a breakfast full of starchy carbohydrates or sugar. She ate cereal or waffles, or sweetened yogurt with fruit. Then she waited until dinner to eat again. She would eat a healthy meal, but would snack on corn chips or popcorn afterward. Desserts were a common treat for her—crème brûlée in particular. Sandee ate like this for years, all the while taking probiotic and fiber supplements along with fish oil and digestive enzymes. After all, Sandee is my sister and after many years of working with me, she knows the importance of such supplements.

Sandee had a rude awakening one day when she learned her blood pressure was too high. Afraid she would end up on medications, she wanted to make some changes. I told her that her diet wasn't supporting her gut health. Yes, she was taking supplements to support her gut, but she was still feeding the harmful bacteria in her gut when she snacked on chips and sweets. It was time for a reality check.

Sandee began to implement the three simple rules of my Skinny Gut Diet:

Rule 1: Eat more fat (*healthy* fat) to reduce silent inflammation.

Rule 2: Eat living foods every day to balance your gut.

Rule 3: Eat protein at every meal and snack to eliminate cravings.

She ate more living foods—those foods that contain good bacteria (also called probiotics) and foods that feed good bacteria in the gut. She made sure to eat healthy fats and to minimize bad fats. She limited her sugar intake to 8 to 10 teaspoons daily (not just added and natural sugars, but also the hidden sugar from digested carbohydrates), using my unique Teaspoon Tracker calculation that shows how many total teaspoons of sugar you get from the starchy carbohydrates and sugar you eat. And she ate protein at every meal and snack, which kept her appetite satisfied throughout the day.

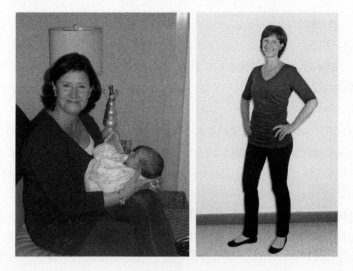

No, that's not her baby!

These dietary changes balanced Sandee's gut and helped her lose 40 pounds in four months. She looked great, but most of all, she felt great. Her blood pressure went down and her energy levels no longer fluctuated in response to her sugar intake. Sandee was happy and relieved that she no longer had to worry about her health. Three years later, Sandee continues to follow the three simple rules of my Skinny Gut Diet and she has kept the weight off—she is as slim today as she was when she first shed those 40 pounds.

THE GUT FACTOR—HOW YOUR BACTERIA MAKE YOU FAT

To understand how your gut bacteria can make you fat, let's take a closer look at the bacteria themselves. There are three types of microbes in your gut: beneficial ("good" or "friendly"), commensal ("neutral"), and potentially pathogenic ("bad" or "harmful"). In general, you want the beneficial microbes to outnumber the potentially pathogenic microbes—the good must outnumber the bad. This is what I mean when I refer to *gut balance*. When the gut is in balance, the potential pathogens will not get the chance to reach pathogenic status. The good bacteria far outnumber the potentially harmful bacteria, keeping them in check by crowding them out and working with the immune system so their numbers stay down. Imagine that inside of you are enough bacteria to form a mass the size of a brick—four pounds. That's right—the bacteria in your gut weigh four pounds. That's a lot of bacteria.

A disturbance of the gut bacterial balance, a condition commonly known as *dysbiosis*, can occur as a result of a number of factors and has been linked to a laundry list of health conditions. From autism and arthritis to heart disease, diabetes, and of course, obesity, an imbalance of gut microbes has been linked to as many conditions outside the gut as inside the gut.

Over the past 25 years, the prevalence of obesity in the United States has increased by more than 75 percent. Nearly two-thirds of the U.S. population is overweight and 1 in 3 adults are clinically obese.

Good Bacteria = Fewer Calories

The gut bacterial composition of obese people differs from that of lean people.[1] Importantly, this difference not only is the *result* of being fat or of eating an obesity-inducing diet but also plays a *causative* role in weight gain. That is, having the wrong balance of bacteria in your gut can make you fat. And having the right balance of gut bacteria can protect you from getting fat. That friend of yours who never gains weight, no matter what she eats? She likely has the right gut bacteria. Your other friend who gains weight despite her efforts to lose it? She may have the wrong bugs in her belly.

It turns out that the gut bacteria of obese people are more efficient at extracting calories from food passing through the digestive tract. When undigested food reaches the colon, or the large intestine, hungry bacteria feast on these foods, harvesting extra calories that are absorbed and added to the body's calorie intake and fat storage. This increased energy intake and fat buildup equals increased weight. So if

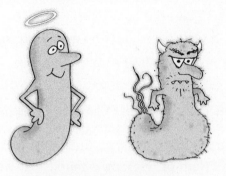

Good Bacteria; Bad Bacteria

two people are fed the exact same diet, but one of them harbors the "obese microbes" (Fat bacteria)—the bacteria found most commonly in obese people—and the other person is lucky enough to house the "lean microbes" (Be Skinny bacteria), then you can guess who gains weight and who doesn't. I don't know about you, but I'll take some of those lean microbes, please.

Gut Type—Lean or Obese?

The majority of gut bacteria make up two main groups (phyla)—Bacteroidetes and Firmicutes. Remember from the Introduction that Firmicutes is the Fat bacteria and Bacteroidetes is the Be Skinny bacteria. An individual's ratio of these two bacterial groups determines whether he or she has a "lean gut type" or an "obese gut type" (a balanced or imbalanced gut). The lean gut type consists of more Be Skinny bacteria and less Fat bacteria than the obese gut type. In a study done by Jeffrey Gordon's lab, a leading research center on the cutting edge of this field, located at Washington University in St. Louis, overweight individuals consumed a weight-loss diet for one year. At the beginning of the study, the participants' ratio of Fat bacteria to Be Skinny bacteria was considerably higher than that of normal weight controls.[2] The overweight people had higher amounts of Fat bacteria and lower amounts of Be Skinny bacteria than their lean counterparts. In those people who were able to lose weight and keep it off up to a year later, the ratio returned to that found in normal weight subjects. Simply put, those who were successful at keeping the weight off had the right bacteria in their guts.

The Discovery That Changed Everything

It all began with a study by Jeffrey Gordon's lab at Washington University. Gordon's team of researchers found that when they put the gut microbes of normal mice into the digestive tracts of mice raised to be *germ free* (without any microbes), the germ-free mice experienced

POOP SCOOP

In a study by Harvard researchers, the gut microbe composition of European children (who eat the same Western diet as American children) was compared to that of children from a rural African village of Burkina Faso, who eat a diet very high in fiber and plant-based foods—living foods.[3] The rural African children had a higher amount of Be Skinny bacteria and lower Fat bacteria, reminiscent of the "lean gut type." The African children also had higher amounts of intestinal health-promoting metabolites produced by good bacteria than did the European children. The researchers concluded that the enrichment of good bacteria found in the African children protected them from inflammation and disease of the colon, and it was the result of their high-fiber diet.

Once again, we see that diet plays a strong role in the development of gut balance. By eating a diet full of living foods—foods that contain good bacteria, and fiber that feeds the good bacteria—you will increase your amount of the beneficial bacteria that are characteristic of the "lean gut type."

a 60 percent increase in body fat and insulin resistance within two weeks.[4] This was the first clue that gut microbes could be responsible for fat accumulation.

This groundbreaking study led to a burgeoning interest in the effects of gut bacteria on obesity and related conditions. The researchers had shown that gut imbalance was not just a *result* of being obese but also that it could be the *cause* of being obese. This discovery was a game-changer. The same researchers followed this pivotal study with another one that confirmed those results.[5] This time, when they transferred the gut microbes from conventionally raised, genetically obese mice into the digestive tracts of germ-free mice, the germ-free mice became obese when compared to a control group of germ-free mice that did not receive microbes. They found that, despite both groups' eating the same diet, the mice that had received the "obese microbes" absorbed more calories than the control group.

What is it about gut microbes that makes them more likely to absorb calories and store fat? Gordon's lab found that the obese mice had a 50 percent reduction in the abundance of Bacteroidetes (Be Skinny) bacteria and a proportional increase in Firmicutes (Fat) bacteria.[6] As you have already learned, these are the main bacteria groups that have been associated with leanness or obesity in humans. It all started with Gordon's lab.

Why run the tests on mice, you might ask? Because studying these effects in humans is more difficult, owing to the many confounding factors, including varied diets, differing lifestyles, and genetic differences. Although we are not mice, fortunately for us mice contain surprisingly similar gut microbes to ours. In fact, when you insert human microbes into a mouse, they colonize as if they were right at home. So in many ways, using mice as models to study the effects of gut microbes on human health is a great starting point for figuring out just what is going on in there.

Scientists can then follow the mouse studies with human studies to determine which of these effects translate to humans. As you have noted, human studies have found that obese adults have lower amounts of Be Skinny bacteria, higher amounts of Fat bacteria, and lower overall bacterial diversity than lean people.[7] For instance, in a study of adolescents, weight loss accompanied an increase in Be Skinny bacteria. And a higher Fat : Be Skinny ratio has also been found in obese children when compared to their lean counterparts.[8]

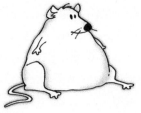

Put simply, the guts of obese people are out of balance. By rebalancing your gut, you can absorb fewer calories from the food you eat. Not a bad deal, huh?

POOP SCOOP

With the right bacteria you can absorb fewer calories. That's right: by changing your gut bacterial composition from an obese profile to a lean profile, you will naturally absorb fewer calories from food. But I want to let you in on another secret. When you eat a diet high in fiber, as you will on the Skinny Gut Diet, you will also absorb fewer calories. Fiber actually helps you reduce absorption of calories from food you have already consumed. As it turns out, people who eat diets high in fiber excrete more calories in their stool. I know this is not a pleasant subject to discuss, but the technical term for this is *fecal energy extraction.* I call it the "fiber flush effect."

Researchers have found that the number of calories excreted from a high-fiber diet equal 10 percent or more of the calories consumed during a given day.[9] Of all the studies done to show the flush effect of fiber on consumed calories, the most thought-provoking one determined that, for every gram of fiber you eat, you eliminate between 8.46 and 12.84 calories.[10] When you do the math and take a conservative average of what various labs have calculated, it's reasonable to say that for every gram of fiber you consume, about 7 calories get eliminated from stool. That means that if you eat a high-fiber diet that consists of 35 grams of fiber daily, you will eliminate 245 calories per day.

You might be wondering how fiber manages to grab calories and rake them out of your body before they become a part of you. The mechanism is actually quite simple. The fiber is blocking the absorption of calories consumed, much like an escort that leads those calories out of your body. The flush effect is just one of fiber's many wonders, as you will learn in this book.

Good Bacteria = Less Fat

Our gut bacteria respond quickly to changes in our diet. Good gut bacteria thrive on certain fibers while bad gut bacteria thrive on diets high in sugar, processed carbohydrates, and unhealthy fats. Well, guess what? The Standard American Diet (SAD) is high in starchy carbohydrates, sugar, and unhealthy fats, and it is low in fiber. When you eat the SAD diet, your gut bacterial balance shifts toward an increase in bad bacteria. This shift produces a moderate amount of bacterial toxins. Most people don't realize that bad bacteria in the gut create their own toxins. These toxins are released in the gut, they damage the intestinal lining, and they are absorbed into the blood-stream, where they are discovered by the immune system. Then, in response to these toxins, the immune system sets off a low-grade in-flammatory response (also known as silent inflammation) as a way to rid the body of the toxins—and you get fatter.

The inflammation response to an unhealthy meal would normally be considered beneficial under temporary conditions. After all, the immune system responds to that which it sees as unhealthy. The problem is that the Standard American Diet (SAD) is just that—standard. When eaten on a regular basis, the gut bacteria continu-ally release those toxins and the immune system continually responds with silent inflammation.

Bacterial imbalance ➤ Digestive toxins ➤ Leaky Gut ➤ Inflammation ➤ Fat storage

You may be wondering how a digestive toxin in the intestinal tract could have anything to do with the fat accumulating on your hips. To understand how this happens, you need to take a closer look at *leaky gut syndrome*. Here's how it works: A one-cell-thick layer lines your intestinal tract, acting like a screen by separating digestive contents from the rest of your body, letting in smaller molecules like water and

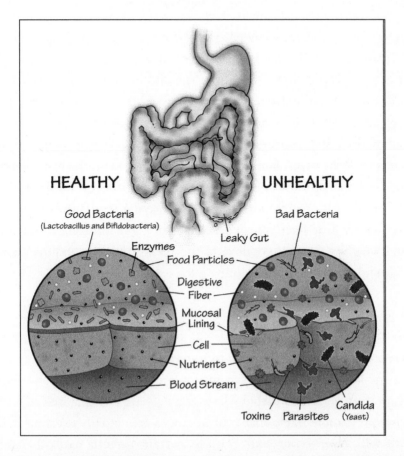

HEALTHY　　　UNHEALTHY

Good Bacteria
(Lactobacillus and Bifidobacteria)　　　Bad Bacteria

Leaky Gut

Enzymes

Food Particles

Digestive Fiber

Mucosal Lining

Cell

Nutrients

Blood Stream

Toxins　Parasites　Candida (Yeast)

nutrients from food and keeping out larger particles like pathogens, undigested food, and toxins. When your gut bacteria are out of balance, the protective lining of the intestines becomes damaged and it can no longer keep out those unwanted particles. Like a hole in your screen door that lets in mosquitoes, suddenly your bloodstream is presented with toxins, pathogens, and undigested food—all considered foreign particles to the body. The immune system responds accordingly by launching a defensive attack that produces inflammation.[11] This inflammation triggers a number of defensive responses by the body that lead to fat storage and weight gain. As gut inflammation increases, you get fatter.

The Standard American Diet, high in fat and sugar, increases the amount of the toxin-producing bacteria and decreases the amount of a particular beneficial gut bacteria known as Bifidobacteria. (You'll learn more about the wonders of Bifidobacteria in Chapter 4.) This decrease in Bifidobacteria also triggers silent inflammation and leads to obesity. Fortunately, increasing the Bifidobacteria in your gut—vital to digestive balance—by taking probiotics and prebiotics has been found to protect against increases in bacterial toxins and inflammation, and to decrease the metabolic dysfunction that leads to obesity.[12] When you change the way you eat to starve the bad bacteria and feed the good bacteria, you can lower your levels of fat storage and reverse the weight gain. So what I'm saying here is that by eating the Skinny Gut Diet you will reverse your gut imbalance and stop your weight gain. Say goodbye to those extra pounds and love handles, and say hello to your skinny gut.

Good Bacteria = Fewer Cravings

Some of the biggest obstacles to implementing a new way of eating are the food cravings that accompany a new diet. While you might think your sugar and carbohydrate cravings are due to a lack of willpower, it is more likely that your microbes are actually exerting their own willpower—over you! You see, certain bacteria and other microbes feed on sugars, using them as a fuel source to reproduce and thrive. Researchers say that *our bacteria may be capable of manipulating our behavior and our appetite in order to obtain more of the sugars they thrive on.*[13]

Remember that our bacteria play a larger role on our health than we generally realize. The gut is connected directly to the brain, both receiving and sending messages to and from that central powerhouse all the time. In fact, the gut is known as the "second brain" because it houses the enteric nervous system within the lining of the digestive tract. This second nervous system consists of about five hundred million neurons—more neurons than in the spinal cord itself. Research has shown that gut bacteria can actually affect your *mental* health. (In Chapter 6, I go into more detail about the gut-brain connection, and how gut bacteria affect mood and behavior.) Let's take a closer look at how gut bacteria can affect an important aspect of your behavior—your appetite.

Candida—the Craving Culprit

One microbe in particular is well known for triggering sugar and carbohydrate cravings—*Candida albicans,* or Candida, for short. Candida is a yeast (a type of fungus), not a bacteria. It resides in the gut, in small numbers, in 80 percent of us. In healthy people, Candida exists in a harmless, unicellular yeast-like form, feeding on sugars and being kept in check by the good bacteria in the gut. But when the gut becomes imbalanced (I'll tell you how in the next chapter), Candida thrives, increasing in number and changing from yeast to a multicellular filamentous form with rootlike structures called hyphae. These hyphae can pierce the intestinal lining, increasing a leaky gut and allowing Candida to enter the bloodstream and reach other tissues in the body.

Candida overgrowth is not a well-recognized condition in conventional medicine, with the exception of vaginal yeast infections and oral thrush (which are Candida overgrowths). Candida overgrowth in the digestive tract, however, is well known to integrative physicians, most commonly occurring after antibiotic use. Antibiotics kill bacteria—the good and the bad—but they do not kill yeast. So Candida is particularly well positioned to flourish after the antibiotics have wiped out the majority of bacteria in the gut. With no competition, Candida feasts on all the sugars and carbohydrates it wants, increasing your cravings for these foods. If you have ever experienced a yeast infection after taking antibiotics, you are familiar with the wrath of Candida.

It's important for you to know that Candida thrives not only in the vaginal tract but also in the digestive tract. In fact, Candida is most at home in the intestines. It is there that Candida has greatest access to its food source—sugar. And the more sugar it has, the more it can grow. One of the most common symptoms in people with Candida overgrowth is sugar cravings. The more you crave sugar, the more sugar you are likely to eat, the more sugar Candida eats. The result is an accelerating cycle of Candida overgrowth and cravings.

> **"Before the Skinny Gut Diet I never realized how much of my diet contained so many carbs. My meals were fairly healthy, but my snacks were all sugar based. I also have realized that I am an emotional eater. Being on the food plan has helped me to slow down, think, and pay attention to what I am eating." —Shirley**

In order to get control over your cravings, you will need to balance your gut with good bacteria so that Candida and other sugar-loving potential pathogens are kept under control. The Skinny Gut Diet will help you do just that. When your gut is in balance, you will notice your cravings disappear. Those urges that once drove you to the snack cupboard multiple times a day will no longer hold you captive. On the Skinny Gut Diet you will find that you prefer foods that nourish your body and not your bad bugs.

Cravings Linked to the Bacteria in Your Mouth

Like the rest of your digestive system, your mouth also plays an important role in your overall health. It has been estimated that 1 trillion bacteria are swallowed with saliva from the mouth each day, helping to "seed" the bacteria in the gut. Researchers from The Forsythe Institute, an epicenter of biotechnology affiliated with Harvard School of Dental Medicine, have hypothesized that oral bacteria may be, at least in part, responsible for initiating obesity.[14] They say that, because all gut bacteria originally pass through the mouth, gut imbalance may actually originate in the mouth. They also suggest that oral bacteria could increase weight gain by increasing appetite; that is, when you eat more, your bacteria get more to eat, too (bacteria eat the food that passes through the digestive tract). In this way, your

POOP SCOOP: FIBER AND THE ANTI-HUNGER HORMONE

What most people don't know is that your small intestine produces a hormone that creates a feeling of fullness. It's cholecystokinin (kol-eh-SIS-toh-kine-in), abbreviated CCK. Think of cholecystokinin as a messenger that tells you, "Okay, I'm full now. I'm not hungry anymore, so put down the fork." What a great messenger to have on your weight-loss team. Well, as it turns out, fiber promotes and prolongs the elevation of CCK in the blood, and these elevated levels make you feel full longer.

Cholecystokinin is a gastrointestinal hormone that's responsible for stimulating the digestion of fat and protein. It is secreted by the first segment of your small intestine, the duodenum, which then causes the release of enzymes from the pancreas and bile from the gallbladder to aid in digestion. In fact, CCK mediates a number of physiological processes, and the good news about this hormone is that it suppresses hunger. It's what helps you push your chair away from the table without feeling deprived. (You will learn more about this effect in Chapter 11.)

bacteria may be able to influence your appetite in order to get more food for themselves. Finally, researchers at the Institute think that oral bacteria may promote obesity by triggering inflammation in the same way as gut bacteria do. Next time you have a food craving, remember that your gut bacteria could be to blame.

Lessons from Gastric Bypass

Currently, the only effective treatment for the most severe form of obesity—morbid obesity—is weight-loss surgery, also called bariatric surgery. The most commonly performed weight-loss surgery is Roux-en-Y gastric bypass, in which the stomach is made smaller and part of the small intestine is bypassed. The individual feels full after eating

SKINNY GUT SUCCESS STORY: POLLY B.

I met Polly at the birthday party of a dear, mutual friend. An acclaimed international speaker and author, Polly was dynamic, enthusiastic, and charming. There was one problem—Polly had battled weight her entire adult life, resulting in her decision for lap band surgery (gastric banding). Laparoscopic gastric banding surgery involves wrapping a device around the upper stomach to make it smaller so that feelings of fullness occur much earlier in the meal than normal. Initially the surgery was successful, but over time it failed miserably, creating severe health problems. As I began talking with Polly, it became clear that she wanted to live a vibrant, healthy life. I let her know that in order to get there she would have to address her digestion.

Before Polly began the Skinny Gut Diet, she was vomiting after meals on a daily basis. She lived in a world of dread and nausea. As a public figure, this situation overwhelmed her. Clearly something was badly out of balance in her gut. Yet her doctors were out of options.

Polly had made inconsistent attempts to balance her gut with supplements, using a box or two of one product here, a box of something else there. She would "try" probiotics or fiber for a month or so, but she failed to implement a complete program that addressed her overall digestion. This is a common practice, unfortunately. When people do not experience a healing miracle after taking one bottle of supplements, they give up. Or, in some cases, people are missing a piece of the puzzle—whether it's another supplement to complete the program or the incorporation of healthy eating habits (or both)—and they see only mild improvements in their health. As a result, they become less interested in supplements as a tool for health transformation.

Gut health is not a fluke. It's the product of good, quality food choices on a daily basis, along with appropriate digestive supplementation. It's not a mystery, but it does take a willingness to understand basic digestive principles and a commitment to follow a restoration program for at least a number of months. Ultimately, the goal is to embrace a lifestyle—yes, for life. That why I am sharing the Skinny Gut Diet with you.

"What a difference a happy gut makes!
Until now I didn't know how great my life could be with improved health and a balanced gut." —Polly

By following the Skinny Gut Diet, you will balance your gut, achieve great health, and feel super inside your body. No one wanted to feel good as much as Polly did. She began the Skinny Gut Diet, and to her delight, she was soon no longer vomiting consistently. My primary emphasis was to repopulate her gut with good bacteria and help repair her intestinal lining using high-potency probiotics. I wanted to be sure her food was breaking down as efficiently as possible, so digestive enzymes were also key to her success. We slowly added fiber to help carry out the toxins and feed her beneficial bacteria. In addition, Polly counted her teaspoons of sugar using my unique Teaspoon Tracker calculation, and was able to eliminate sugar cravings that had haunted her for so long.

At 5 foot 4 inches, Polly lost 37 pounds during the three months of the Skinny Gut Diet program, and she continues to lose weight steadily. She completed a 5K walk toward the end of the program that, she said, couldn't have been done without the Skinny Gut Diet. Although most people will not face the extreme health issues that Polly had at the onset of the program, I am grateful to share her journey. It is an inspiring story of hope and success.

a small amount of food and will absorb fewer calories, usually losing 65 to 75 percent of his or her excess weight after the surgery. The changes resulting from altering the digestive tract in this way change the gut bacteria to be more like that found in lean individuals.[15]

Researchers wanted to understand these gut bacterial changes better, so they used an animal model to do so. From two groups of mice—one group that had received gastric bypass and another group that did not—they transplanted gut microbes into germ-free mice. Both groups of recipient mice ate the same diet, but the ones that received microbes from the post-gastric surgery mice lost weight and body fat when compared to the mice that received microbes from mice that did not undergo surgery.[16] Once again, we see the mice that lost weight had increased amounts of Bacteroidetes (Be Skinny bacteria) and decreased amounts of Firmicutes (Fat bacteria). The researchers think they may one day be able to modulate the gut microbes of obese people *without* having to resort to weight-loss surgery. To think, we hold the potential for weight loss within our guts. That's a powerful thought!

In a study in humans (because, let's face it, we aren't mice), people underwent gastric bypass and were given a *Lactobacillus* probiotic to take every day for six months after surgery.[17] The researchers were hoping to find a decrease in bacterial overgrowth, a common side effect of the surgery, in the people taking the probiotic. To their surprise, not only did they find a decrease in bacterial overgrowth, but they also found greater weight loss in the group taking the *Lactobacillus* probiotic when compared to the control group. Given the severity of morbid obesity, these studies sure give us hope.

If You Want to Dig Deeper

By now you have some understanding about how your gut bacteria can make you fat. If you want to delve deeper into the science behind this fascinating phenomenon, see pages 241 to 252 of the Appendix, where Dr. Leonard Smith explains the links between gut imbalance and weight gain. For now, let's keep learning about how gut bacteria get out of balance in the first place.

CHAPTER 2 SUMMARY

Good Bacteria = Fewer Calories
➤ Gut bacteria of obese people extract extra calories from food passing through the digestive tract.
➤ The majority of gut bacteria are made up of two main groups—Bacteroidetes and Firmicutes. An individual's ratio of these two bacterial groups determines whether he or she has a "lean gut type" or an "obese gut type" (a balanced or imbalanced gut).

Good Bacteria = Less Fat
➤ Gut imbalance leads to silent inflammation, which triggers a number of responses in the body that result in fat storage and weight gain.

Good Bacteria = Fewer Cravings
➤ Candida overgrowth may be responsible for your sugar and carb cravings. Keeping Candida in check by balancing your gut will help eliminate these cravings.

Chapter 3

WHERE DID IT ALL GO WRONG?

Gut bacterial balance functions like an ecosystem. It's a community of living organisms that all depend on each other in some way. In an ecosystem, when one species is removed, an invasive species might overtake a habitat, crowding out the species that previously had thrived there. In the digestive system this type of organism is known as an *opportunistic pathogen*, like Candida and the harmful bacteria mentioned earlier. Normally existing peacefully in small numbers, an opportunistic pathogen will gain the upper hand when other, beneficial bacteria are depleted. Maintaining a healthy balance of gut bacteria is crucial not only for weight loss but also for keeping peace in your gut.

At birth, or shortly thereafter, you were inoculated with bacteria. If you were birthed traditionally, down the vaginal canal, your mother passed on her bacteria to you, at which point they began to colonize and multiply on your skin. You swallowed some of these bacteria and they colonized your digestive tract, concentrating in the intestines.

If you were born vaginally, and thus colonized by bacteria in this way, it turns out you are at a health advantage when it comes to being protected against infection, allergies, and immune dysfunction. The development of a healthy balance of gut microbes consisting of a diverse range of bacteria is important for infant health and the proper development of the intestines and immune system, which set the stage for a healthy life. Inoculation by the right microbes at birth gives you a one-up, so to speak, on your health.

If you were born by Cesarean section, however, you came into the world with a microbial handicap, according to what researchers are discovering. Children who are born via C-section are colonized by a much different mix of bacteria. They inherit, to a greater extent than vaginally born infants, the environmental microbes from the air, and from the skin and mouths of their mothers, as well as from the skin of hospital staff, resulting in fewer intestinal *Bifidobacterium* and *Bacteroides* species (both protective against obesity) and more *Clostridium difficile* (a pathogenic bacteria).[1] Babies born by Cesarean also have a slower-developing diversity of gut bacteria than babies born vaginally,[2] and those bacteria more closely resemble bacteria commonly found on skin rather than bacteria found in a healthy gut.

> **According to the Centers for Disease Control, one-third of births in the United States are by Cesarean section.**

Researchers investigating the link between gut bacteria and health wanted to know if early gut bacterial composition could predict the later development of obesity. Could it be that the childhood obesity epidemic is fueled, in part, by a bacterial imbalance in the guts of infants? Researchers from Finland set out to find the answer to that question. They compared stool samples from overweight or obese children to those of normal-weight children, and they discovered significantly higher numbers of Bifidobacteria in the infants who ended up normal weight at seven years, when compared to those children who ended up overweight.[3] Bifidobacteria are well known for providing a number of benefits to the host (that's you!), including reduced gut inflammation or leaky gut, healthy gut lining, production of beneficial metabolites, and improved immune function. Not only did the researchers find lower amounts of Bifidobacteria in the children who later developed obesity, but they also found higher amounts of *Staphylococcus aureus*. They proposed that *S. aureus* triggers low-grade inflammation, leading to the development of obesity.[4] Once again, gut imbalance and silent inflammation are tied to obesity.

Another study by the same Finnish researchers found that gut microbe composition differs between overweight and normal-weight pregnant women.[5] What's more, the gut bacteria not only contribute to weight gain in pregnant mothers but also predict the later development of obesity in children born to these mothers. It's another vicious cycle: gut imbalance contributes to weight gain during pregnancy; the mothers then pass the bacteria on to their infants, who later become overweight and those overweight children are more likely to become overweight adults. This cycle surely helps explain the current obesity epidemic, doesn't it?

Fortunately, there is a backup system for improving the balance of gut bacteria during infancy—nature's perfect food, *breast milk*. Breast milk contains the perfect nutrition for babies, as long as the mother is well nourished. The unique nutritional qualities of breast milk have not always been appreciated, however. An abundance of indigestible material called *oligosaccharides* in the breast milk puzzled researchers for decades. Oligosaccharides are a type of soluble fiber, the presence of which, given their nonnutritive properties, seemed a paradox. Why would breast milk contain these oligosac-

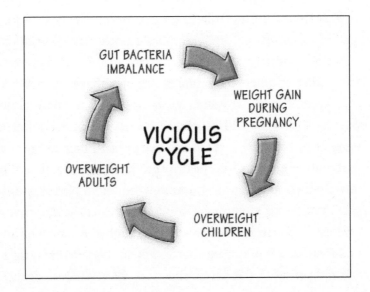

charides if they are not absorbed as nutrients by the infant? As it turns out, these soluble fibers act as food for a good gut bacterium found in the healthy guts of infants: *Bifidobacterium infantis*. Breast milk itself also contains a number of Bifidobacteria, including *B. longum, B. animalis, B. bifidum,* and *B. catenulatum.*[6] Bifidobacteria produce beneficial compounds that nourish the intestinal lining and help keep potential pathogens at bay. In general, the more Bifidobacteria in your gut, the better your bacterial balance. If you were breast-fed for at least six months, you were lucky enough to establish a healthy gut balance rich in Bifidobacteria. Unfortunately, other factors may have interfered with maintaining this balance, as you will learn.

Before you begin to fret that your gut bacteria are destined for imbalance because of factors surrounding your birth and upbringing, rest assured that you can bring balance to your gut with probiotics and the right diet. The Skinny Gut Diet will show you how.

The Human Microbiome Project

The Human Microbiome Project is a massive research initiative funded by the National Institutes of Health (NIH). It began in 2008 with the mission of identifying and characterizing the human microbiome—the collection of microbes, including bacteria, living in and on the human body, along with their DNA—to determine its role in human health and disease. Involving eighty universities and scientific institutions, the research project has defined the normal human microbiome of healthy Westerners and has begun to investigate how the microbiome is associated with human health and disease.

Researchers found, for example, that almost everyone harbors potential pathogens—microorganisms that are known to cause disease. In healthy people, these pathogens are kept in check by the beneficial bacteria that reside in the same vicinity. That is, the gut bacteria collectively maintain a balance so that those pathogens cannot thrive.

The importance of maintaining this balance, then, becomes obvious when you understand that your very health is at stake. In other words, your health is not so much under your control as under the control of your bacteria.

"Disorders in our internal ecosystem—a loss of diversity, say, or a proliferation of the 'wrong' kind of microbes—may predispose us to obesity and a whole range of chronic diseases, as well as some infections."

—Michael Pollan, "Some of Our Best Friends Are Germs," New York Times, May 15, 2013

The Human Microbiome Project found that healthy people have a more diverse mix of microbes. This diversity is thought to be a cornerstone of human health, just as it is a cornerstone of a healthy ecosystem. "It appears bacteria can pinch-hit for each other," stated Curtis Huttenhower, one of the researchers. In baseball, pinch hitters are substitute batters who have a better chance of reaching base or scoring than the batters they replace. Likewise, different bacteria can perform similar functions, replacing each other when needed. For example, many species of bacteria produce butyrate, a short-chain fatty acid (SCFA) that feeds the intestinal lining, which helps make new cells and heal a leaky gut. When you eat a diet high in fiber and you have the right bacteria in your gut, your bacteria will produce beneficial SCFAs. This is just one of many ways that bacteria work together to promote health (or, if the wrong microbes are dominant and the diet is low in fiber, to promote disease).

Good bacteria + fiber ➤ Butyrate (SCFA) ➤ Food for colon cells

TOO CLEAN FOR OUR OWN GOOD?

The modern world has developed medical practices that have increased life expectancy in the United States by over twenty years since 1900.[7] No doubt, the discovery of penicillin in the early nineteenth century has largely been responsible for such a big jump in longevity. This development, paired with sanitation practices that are the hallmark of contemporary medicine, has provided us with ultra-clean environments that are scrubbed as germ free as possible. From our antibacterial soaps and hand sanitizers to chlorine-spiked cleansers and wipes, concern about germs has taken us from a society living off the bacteria-laden land to one that is a virtual bubble of cleanliness.

Although this relatively recent change in living environment has helped us gain years of life, researchers say that it has come with some health setbacks. According to the *hygiene hypothesis*, a medical rationale proposed in 1989 by epidemiologist David Strachan, children who are raised in "less clean" environments—such as in developing countries, where children play in the dirt and are exposed more to animals (and thus microbes), and where hand sanitizer is generally reserved for medical use—are much less likely to develop allergic conditions like asthma and eczema.[8] The reason for this is that early exposure to a diverse array of microbes primes the immune system so that it can later recognize potential allergens as harmless. In fact, another group of experts proposes an alternate interpretation of the hygiene hypothesis, renaming it the *microflora hypothesis* for its recognition of the integral role played by the gut bacteria.[9] Thus, it is felt that early exposure to everyday bacteria helps balance the immune system. And a balanced immune system is the hallmark of good health.

"Under an evolutionary perspective, the obesity epidemic can be viewed as an extension of the hygiene hypothesis: the data presented suggest that improved sanitation and living conditions, overzealous antimicrobial therapy, and Westernized dietary patterns in developed countries may predispose to metabolic diseases just as improved hygiene increased the susceptibility to allergic and autoimmune disease, and that a deviant gut microbiota may mediate these associations."[10]

ANTIBIOTICS—THE DOUBLE-EDGED SWORD

In line with the hygiene hypothesis, it is believed that overuse of antibiotics is a major contributor to altered gut balance. In fact, antibiotics are part of what has contributed to the hygiene hypothesis. The word *antibiotic* means "against life." Antibiotics destroy not only harmful bacteria but also beneficial bacteria. These drugs alter the gut bacterial composition so much that some researchers state it can never fully return to its previous state.[11] At best, it takes weeks or even months to reestablish the balance, during which time any number of health conditions may arise owing to a compromised gut balance.

For example, if you were born via the birth canal and breast-fed for at least six months, yet you received antibiotics at some point (and who hasn't?)—and especially if you have received multiple courses of antibiotics—your gut bacterial balance has been compromised. This is what happened to me. I was given many antibiotics as a child and I suffered for it with chronic constipation—a clear indication of gut imbalance. But who knew? If your childhood was like most children in the developed world, you received between ten and twenty courses of antibiotics by the time you were 18 years old, and many of those antibiotics were given during your first five years of life. Antibiotic use during infancy lowers the amount of beneficial Bifidobacteria in the gut, resulting in dysbiosis (an imbalance of good and bad bacteria) at an early, delicate age.[12]

Antibiotic use is a major, controllable cause of gut imbalance, and, yes, it is thought to be contributing to the obesity epidemic.

The implications of this connection are enormous, given the widespread use of antibiotics and the prevalence of obesity. Antibiotic use during infancy—particularly during the first six months—has been linked to increased risk of obesity later in life.[13] Part of this problem, though, is the *overuse* of antibiotics. Infants and children (and adults, for that matter) who visit their doctors with an ear infection, sore throat, or cough are usually given a prescription for antibiotics. There is one problem, however: most of the time these infections are *viral*, not bacterial, in origin. Antibiotics kill bacteria, not viruses, so the antibiotics are being prescribed for a condition they do not even treat.[14]

Previously, experts thought that gut bacteria recovered within a few weeks after antibiotic use, but recent studies have found that is not the case. In two recent studies, researchers investigating the effects of the antibiotic ciprofloxacin for a period of eight to ten months following treatment found permanent alterations in gut bacteria.[15] In one study, the gut bacterial composition resembled its pretreatment state after four weeks, with the exception of several bacteria groups that did not recover even six months later. In the second study, the gut bacterial composition finally stabilized after ten months, but differed from its original state. The investigators concluded, "Antibiotic [disruption] may cause a shift to an alternative stable state, the full consequences of which remain unknown."

In another study, the long-term effects of two antibiotics—clarithromycin and metronidazole—were investigated over a four-year period. Although the diversity of gut bacteria subsequently recovered to resemble the pretreatment states, in some people the microbial balance remained altered for up to four years after treatment. Four years! And some researchers say that after the effects of antibiotics, the gut bacteria may never fully recover to their previous state. Yet another study, this of people who took the antibiotic clindamycin for seven days, found persistent long-term impacts on the intestinal bacteria that remained during the two years of that study.[16]

Given everything I've mentioned to now, you can see why antibiotics can be a problem. Clearly, antibiotics are reshaping our gut eco-systems, which experts believe is having widespread negative effects.

Antibiotic Use Linked to Obesity

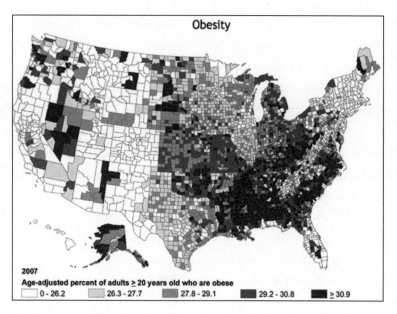

Centers for Disease Control and Prevention, "County-Specific Diabetes and Obesity Prevalence," Morbidity and Mortality Weekly Report, *2007*

The diagrams on this and the next page show the obesity rates (above) and antibiotic use (next page) across the United States in 2007. Did you notice that the maps look strikingly similar? Antibiotic use has been regionally correlated to obesity—the states with the highest obesity rates also exhibit the highest antibiotic use, and the least obese states use the least antibiotics. Coincidence? I don't think so.

Antibiotics are well known to increase body weight in animals. In fact, 70 percent of all the antibiotics sold in the United States are used in livestock farming—eight times the rate of use in human medicine. The widespread use of antibiotics on farms is, for the most part, not to prevent illness in the animals but, rather, to fatten them up. In the 1950s, not long after the first ones were discovered, antibiotics were approved for agricultural use to help prevent disease epidemics. Farmers began to notice that those animals receiving antibiotics gained more weight than the animals not taking the drugs. Fatter, heavier livestock fetch a higher price, so it didn't take long for widespread implementation of low-dose antibiotic feeding of poultry, cattle, and swine. Interestingly, the younger the animals are when the antibiotic feeding is begun, the greater is the weight gain.[17]

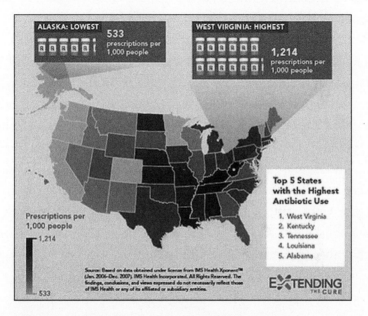

© The Center for Disease Dynamics, Economics & Policy; cddep.org

Translated to humans, this observation suggests that early alteration of the gut bacteria is a particular risk factor for development of obesity. It sheds light on what antibiotics during childhood might be doing to our children. Dr. Martin Blaser, Director of the NYU Human Microbiome Project, asked, "Given that this manipulation of the microbiota has such effects on early life energy homeostasis [balance] and body mass development in farm animals, what might the effects be of the widespread exposure of children to antibiotics early in life?"[18] Indeed.

Dr. Blaser set out to find the answer to this question by creating two animal models: one that mimicked the low-dose administration of antibiotics as received by farm animals and another that mimicked the short, high-dose pulses of antibiotics as received by children. In the first model, those mice that received low-dose antibiotics via drinking water experienced increased fat accumulation, altered gut bacterial balance, and a change in fat and carbohydrate metabolism when compared to control mice. In the second model, those mice that received pulsed antibiotic treatment gained more weight and had an altered bacterial balance compared to control mice.[19]

"We speculate that the widespread treatment of young children with antibiotics has caused alterations in the compositions of their intestinal microbiota, and the luminal signals to the host, that are directly contributing to the epidemic of obesity in developed countries," he stated. "Intensive early-life antibiotic use among human children may similarly contribute to trends in growth by altering the microbiome." The increase in weight experienced in farm animals is due to changes in the gut bacteria induced by the antibiotics, as researchers from the University of Illinois at Urbana-Champaign reported in a study published in 2002.[20] Essentially, their guts are out of balance, which makes them fat. Sound familiar?

The use of antibiotics for growth in agriculture has come under intense scrutiny for its contribution to the development of *antibiotic resistance,* or the resistance of bacteria to commonly used antibiotics. Antibiotic resistance is one of the major challenges facing modern medicine. When antibiotics no longer work against the pathogens that produce disease, we will be back at square one when it comes to treating infections. It seems we have been taking the mighty antibiotic for granted. The Food and Drug Administration (FDA) has asked pharmaceutical companies to voluntary stop selling antibiotics as livestock growth promoters, but the voluntary nature of this request suggests that the solution is not a strong enough measure. In contrast, most European countries have banned the use of antibiotics for growth stimulation in agriculture. The dire consequences of this

GUT SCIENCE WITH DR. LEONARD SMITH

Antibiotic Resistance

Antibiotic resistance is the ability of bacteria to survive in the presence of antibiotics. In any group of bacteria, there are usually a few individual bacteria cells that are resistant to antibiotics. These few bacteria survive in the presence of antibiotics and reproduce to form a new colony that includes more antibiotic-resistant bacteria than the last. If another round of antibiotics is given, this larger number of resistant bacteria will survive and reproduce to form an even larger resistant colony. You can see that the risk of antibiotic resistance increases with each course of antibiotics taken, as the number of resistant bacteria increases.

A recent report on the global effects of antibiotic resistance warns that "we are at the dawn of a post-antibiotic era," with "almost all disease-causing bacteria resistant to the antibiotics commonly used to treat them."[21] The gravity of the problem has been summed up in a commentary of the report: "Rarely has modern medicine faced such a grave threat. Without antibiotics, treatments from minor surgery to major transplants could become impossible," and "infection-related mortality rates in developed countries might return to those of the early 20th century."[22]

The global burden of resistance is probably concentrated in three major categories:

1. Longer duration of illness and higher death rates in patients with resistant infections.
2. Increasing costs of treatment for resistant infections.
3. Inability to perform procedures (i.e., surgeries) that rely on antibiotics to prevent infection.

Sadly, this message is not new. In fact, back in 1945, Sir Alexander Fleming warned of the danger of antibiotic resistance resulting from overuse of antibiotics. Yet here we are almost seventy years later, still largely ignoring this advice.

The report just cited calls for a national commitment, on a global scale, to implement successful strategies for "getting out of the impasse." The researchers ask for rational use of antibiotics in hospitals and in the community. They imply a need for changes in education and social norms. (The attitude, "But I always take/prescribe antibiotics for a cough/sore throat/cold/urinary tract infection/acne/etc." must change if we are to reverse the trend.) They call for better diagnostics, elimination of inappropriate antibiotic use in agriculture, new antibiotics, and alternative strategies to treat existing and future antibiotic-resistant infections. "The future of antibiotics and survival of every human being that acquires a bacterial infection will depend on the serious commitment of many stakeholders, including government authorities, policy makers, health-care workers, university teachers, pharmaceutical companies, and consumers," they warn.[23]

The judicious use of antibiotics is crucial not only at the global population level but also at the individual level. If you take antibiotics frequently, your bacteria gradually become more resistant to those antibiotics, and one day you will find that the antibiotic that always worked for you suddenly will not. Then you will have to take a broad-spectrum antibiotic, which targets a broader range of bacteria. But the more you take broad-spectrum antibiotics, the more likely a broad range of your gut bacteria will become resistant. Do you see the vicious cycle here?

According to the Centers for Disease Control (CDC), "nearly 2 million people in the United States acquire an infection while in a hospital, resulting in 90,000 deaths. More than 70 percent of the bacteria that cause these infections are resistant to at least one of the antibiotics commonly used to treat them." Antibiotic-resistant infections themselves affect more than 2 million people each year, of which more than 23,000 die as a result.[24]

So, we are now basically being forced back to the natural order of things, in which bacteria fight bacteria. With healthy, flexible immune balance—achieved through a preventive health-care program that includes prebiotics, probiotics, fermented foods and beverages, a diet rich in nonstarchy vegetables and low-sugar fruits, optimum amounts of healthy omega-3 fats, vitamin D3, vitamin C, zinc, selenium, magnesium, and immune-boosting mushrooms along with stress reduction, exercise, adequate sleep, and regular elimination—most people will likely survive serious infections.

New solutions are required that can address the disruption of the microbiome that has come from overuse of antibiotics. Let's fast-forward to the logical and natural biological solution. Pharmaceutical companies will create super probiotics with 50 to 200 strains offering a broad spectrum of action against pathogenic bacteria and fungi. These super probiotics will help fight infections by maintaining a healthy microbiome. There will be specific, individual strains of microbes used to treat specific infections.

An example of the latter that's been in use for over fifteen years is the probiotic yeast *Saccharomyces boulardii,* which suppresses or kills *Clostridium difficile* bacteria. The *C. difficile* diarrhea that results from overuse of broad-spectrum antibiotics can lead to removal of a severely inflamed colon, or even death. But fecal transplants (infusions of beneficial bacteria from stools of healthy donors) have been found to be more than 90 percent effective at wiping out the *C. difficile* infection and healing the patient. The fecal transplants go far beyond fighting *C. difficile,* however. Evidence exists that this technique will be useful also in fighting obesity, insulin resistance (prediabetes), and neurological disorders such as Parkinsonism. Instead of fecal transplants, one day we will have super probiotics that closely parallel the diversity of a healthy microbiome. The world is poised to wake up to recognizing the gut microbiome as the cornerstone of health and longevity.

practice are not yet appreciated in the United States, despite many experts' calls for action.[25]

Additionally, unused antibiotics, or antibiotics that are unmetabolized and excreted in urine, end up in our sewage systems. Oh, my—we are actually peeing out so many antibiotics that they can be measured! Because these drugs are being degraded well or eliminated during sewage treatment, they eventually reach groundwater supplies and potentially enter our drinking water. Plus, the antibiotics excreted in the urine of farm animals, which enter the soil and eventually make their way also into groundwater nearby, compounds the environmental impact of antibiotic use. What about antibiotic residues that make their way into our drinking water? Unfortunately, current research in these areas is scant, despite scientists' concerns.[26]

But wait, there's more. Antibiotic residues can be found in the meat, dairy, and fish we consume, owing to all the antibiotics they receive. Sure, limits are set on the amount of allowable antibiotic residues in these foods, but what is the effect of continual, small antibiotic dosages of these residues on our gut bacteria and our weight?

THE STRESS EFFECT

Most people I meet who are facing health challenges exclaim that they are stressed—stressed at work, stressed with family drama, stressed at being a caregiver. Stress plays a prominent role in virtually everyone's life. From endless to-do lists and extended workdays to responsibilities and deadlines at every turn, we experience chronic stress as the norm in modern life. The detrimental effects of stress are often discussed—poor heart health, emotional upheaval, inability to concentrate, and digestive disruptions—but what you may not have considered is that all that stress has an effect on the balance of your gut bacteria as well.

Connections between decreases in the beneficial bacteria *Lacto-*

bacillus and *Bifidobacterium* and increased susceptibility to infections have been demonstrated in animal studies that have evaluated the effects of stress on the gut. Researchers have also found shifts in the proportions of some gut bacterial species in people experiencing stress from anger or fear. Chronic stress has been found to decrease the abundance of *Bacteroides* bacteria (generally considered beneficial) and increase *Clostridium* bacteria (some are potentially pathogenic) along with inflammation. And emotional stress can lead to long-term reductions in both Lactobacilli and Bifidobacteria.[27] Recent studies support the role of probiotics in alleviating stress-induced alterations of gut function, particularly by reducing intestinal permeability, or leaky gut, which further highlights the importance of gut bacterial balance for people under stress. Bifidobacteria have been found to be extremely sensitive to emotional stress as well as stressful physical demands. In addition to altering the gut bacteria, chronic stress disturbs the intestinal lining, increasing leaky gut and the amount of bacterial toxins in circulation.[28]

Fortunately, probiotics can reverse these effects of stress.[29] In one study, probiotics were found to decrease stress response by preventing the destruction of the intestinal lining and decreasing the amount of circulating bacterial toxins.[30] So, by rebalancing the gut, the harmful effects of stress can be reversed—now that's a stress reliever! In short, by taking probiotics you can lessen the effects of stress on both your body and your mind.

Stress can also contribute to either ulcers or inflammation of the stomach (a condition known as *gastritis*), both of which can cause significant blood loss and, in extreme cases, even death. Stress can decrease blood flow to the stomach, which, combined with nutritional deficiency, weakens the stomach lining, making it susceptible to bleeding independent of stomach acid levels. For these reasons, most doctors put patients suffering these effects on acid blockers to protect the compromised stomach lining, which can then create other serious problems, especially if the stomach acid was already low.

Based on test results, 80 percent of Skinny Gut Diet
participants began the diet with impaired production of
digestive enzymes and poor absorption of nutrients.
All of them experienced vast improvements in digestive
health over the course of the diet.

Stomach acid, also known as *hydrochloric acid,* serves a few very important functions. First, it helps sterilize the stomach, killing off potential pathogens, which consequently helps to prevent gastrointestinal infections. It may sound like killing off all your bacteria is something you wouldn't want to do, given what I have told you about beneficial bacteria, but the stomach is one place where we want to minimize the chance of pathogens getting through.

Additionally, stomach acid helps to denature proteins. Proteins are complex molecules, made up of long strands of amino acids that are twisted and tangled. Hydrochloric acid helps to untangle the strands so that digestive enzymes can access them, breaking down the proteins into absorbable nutrients. Without adequate hydrochloric acids, proteins are not well digested.

Lastly, the presence of hydrochloric acid in the stomach triggers the release of a protein from the stomach lining called *intrinsic factor* that binds to vitamin B12 and assists in the small intestine's absorption of this essential vitamin. Without enough stomach acid, you can develop a B12 deficiency even when your diet contains adequate amounts. B12 is vital for metabolism and neurologic function.

UP WITH YOUR AGE, DOWN WITH YOUR BIFIDO, UP WITH YOUR WEIGHT

With age comes a decline in, well, just about everything—energy levels, mental capacities, libido, you name it. If it's good, or good for you, most likely it declines with age. The same can be said for gut bacteria. Not only does overall gut bacterial diversity decrease, but so do the levels of your beneficial Bifidobacteria. Along with this decrease comes an increase in putrification, or decomposition, in the intestines that increases susceptibility to disease. According to one researcher, "The reduction or disappearance of Bifidobacteria in the human intestine would indicate an 'unhealthy' state."[31]

During infancy, Bifidobacteria levels dominate the intestinal tract; during adulthood, the levels begin to decline but still remain high; and in the senior years, the levels drop significantly. Experts suggest that the decrease in Bifidobacteria occurs due to a reduced ability for the beneficial bacteria to adhere to the intestinal lining.[32] All along the intestinal lining, good bacteria (including Bifidobacteria) create a protective barrier that helps prevent damage to the intestines by pathogens, inflammation, toxins, or other foreign substances. Not only do these bacteria form a physical barrier, but they also create substances that inhibit harmful bacteria. Lactic and acetic acid are both produced by Bifidobacteria and help to maintain a healthy intestinal pH level that inhibits pathogens. In addition, remember that Bifidobacteria also produce short-chain fatty acids that feed the lining of the intestine, fortifying this protective layer.

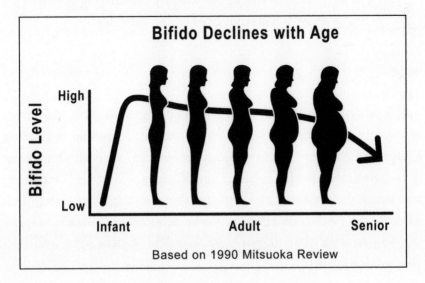

Bifido Declines with Age

Bifido Level

High

Low

Infant   Adult   Senior

Based on 1990 Mitsuoka Review

SKINNY GUT SUCCESS STORY: SHIRLEY J.

Shirley is a truly inspiring woman. At 80 years young, she maintains a full-time accounting position, is a caregiver for her sister, enjoys a great relationship with her daughter, and exercises regularly. Shirley's initial 151 pounds, although not out of control, were weighing her down. At 5 foot 2 inches, the extra pounds felt heavy and ungainly for a woman who had danced most of her life. She had been trying unsuccessfully to lose weight since her heart surgery the previous year, when her doctor advised that the closer she was to a healthy weight for her frame, the less strain she would put on her heart.

Of Italian descent, Shirley clearly loved her pastas, breads, pretzels, and desserts. Although she enjoyed proteins and vegetables at mealtimes, it turns out that Shirley's weakness was high-carbohydrate snacks. As you can imagine, the idea of eliminating carb-heavy crunchy foods and very sweet fruits was less than appealing to her. I have to tell you, Shirley has succeeded.

"I have not had on a belt in at least seven years. I wore my first one this week. I have a waist and much less fat around the belly. Best of all, I've found snacks that are just as satisfying as those chips and pretzels used to be." —Shirley

Maintaining healthy levels of beneficial gut bacteria, therefore, is important for digestive and overall health, including protection against weight gain. Probiotic supplementation with Bifidobacteria is recommended for people over age 50, as a way to help replenish and maintain the beneficial bacteria that are lost with aging. The Skinny Gut Diet is designed to boost Bifidobacteria levels, helping you to maintain your digestive balance and ideal weight well into your golden years.

On the Skinny Gut Diet, Shirley began to observe her eating patterns. Her aha! moment came when she realized that she snacked all day long. She wouldn't even sit down to eat a meal when she was home—she simply chewed and crunched through all her activities. She tells me that the Skinny Gut Diet, by drawing attention to her habits and regulating her eating patterns, has brought her a new appreciation for food and for how much and how often she eats. Now she actually enjoys and tastes what she consumes. And she loves to eat fermented foods—she has no problem snacking on those.

The best news is that Shirley has let go of 11 pounds so far. Her bloating is gone. Her movements are more graceful. She tells me that her thoughts are sharper. It's never too late to make the effort to balance your gut. As Shirley said recently, "Who says you can't teach an old dog new tricks?" Shirley, you are my hero. How great it is that you never stop being willing to learn.

Shirley	Weight	Waistline Inches	Body Fat %
Before	151	36½"	41.4%
After	140	34½"	35.9%
Lost	11 lbs	2"	5.5%

THE MEDICATION SIDE EFFECTS YOUR DOCTOR NEVER TOLD YOU ABOUT

In addition to antibiotics, another commonly used medication—proton pump inhibitors (PPIs)—can cause gut bacterial imbalances that range from inconvenient to fatal. These PPIs are stomach acid–suppressing medications prescribed to more than 15 million people each year for acid reflux (and that doesn't count the millions of people who take over-the-counter versions of the drug). The PPIs work by shutting down the production of stomach acid. This may temporarily ease the symptoms of acid reflux, but stomach acid exists for some very good reasons, as mentioned earlier in the discussion on stress.

First, stomach acid maintains a low pH in the stomach, which inhibits the growth of pathogenic bacteria. When stomach acid is suppressed with PPI use, potential pathogens can more easily through the stomach and enter the intestines, where they proliferate. One particular pathogen—*Clostridium difficile*—has been found to increase with PPI use. *C. difficile* infections affect more than half a million people each year and have become more frequent, severe, fatal, and difficult to treat in recent years.[33]

Proton pump inhibitors (PPIs), also called acid blockers, are commonly used to treat heartburn and acid reflux. PPIs are the third largest-selling drug in the United States. Over 15 million people receive PPI prescriptions annually,[34] generating $14 billion annually—and that doesn't count the millions more who use over-the-counter PPIs on a regular basis. Long-term use of the drug is not recommended, most notably because it leads to gut imbalance and increased risk of infection.

Not only do PPIs affect the intestinal balance, but they have also been found to affect levels of beneficial *Lactobacillus* in the mouth.[35] The digestive tract actually begins in the mouth, and when an imbalance exists in one area of the digestive system, it affects the balance in other areas. Proton pump inhibitors also increase small intestinal bacterial overgrowth (SIBO), a condition in which bacteria from the colon, or large intestine, back up into the small intestine and grow at a rate similar to that of the colon.[36] The small intestine normally contains a lower number of bacteria, so when bacteria overgrow in the small intestine an imbalance, or dysbiosis, results. And, as you have learned, gut imbalance can lead to weight gain.

I need to emphasize that those proton pump inhibitors are not meant for long-term use. (Read the warning on the box if you don't believe me.) And yet, millions of people take these drugs, over the counter or otherwise, on a regular basis; indeed, many take them for years at a time. The result is widespread gut imbalance.

EVERYDAY TOXINS AND GUT HEALTH

There are over 80,000 chemicals currently in use, with 1,000 added each year. We come in contact with hundreds of toxins on a daily basis, many of which have been found to have negative effects on our health. In fact, even infants are born with hundreds of toxins already in their body. A 2005 study by the Environmental Working Group analyzed the umbilical cord blood of ten newborn infants and found 287 industrial chemicals already accumulated.[37] Of those 287 chemicals, 180 are known to cause cancer in humans or animals, 217 are toxic to the brain and nervous system, and 208 cause birth defects or abnormal development in animal models. Sadly, the harmful effects on infants of a chemical cocktail of this sort have never been investigated. Some of the toxins we come into contact with everyday are contributing to digestive imbalance.

If there is one chemical that most of the world is exposed to, it's glyphosate, the active ingredient in the most widely used herbicide worldwide. Although its manufacturer asserts that glyphosate is minimally toxic to humans,[38] some experts disagree. Glyphosate residues are found in the foods on which the herbicide is used, including sugar, corn, soy, and wheat. One of the industry's claims for the safety of glyphosate is that it acts on a certain pathway in plants that does not exist in mammals. This pathway is present in gut bacteria, however, and researchers have found that glyphosate negatively impacts gut bacteria. Glyphosate has been found in animal models to be toxic to beneficial *Lactobacillus, Bifidobacterium,* and *Enterococcus* bacteria while favoring the growth of toxic *Clostridium* species. Further, glyphosate inhibits the function of important detoxification enzymes responsible for the removal of toxins from the body. For these reasons glyphosate has been proposed by some experts as contributing to "most of the diseases and conditions associated with a Western diet, which include gastrointestinal disorders, obesity, diabetes, heart disease, depression, autism, infertility, cancer, and Alzheimer's disease."[39]

Heavy metal toxicity is also a factor that contributes to gut bacterial imbalance. The greatest exposure to heavy metals comes by way of mercury-containing (silver) dental amalgam fillings, which release small amounts of heavy metals over time from the normal wear and tear of chewing. Mercury released from such fillings has been found to increase the antibiotic-resistant oral and intestinal bacteria.[40] Heavy metal exposure can also come from lead paint and lead pipes in older houses that have not been updated. Many integrative health practitioners find that elevated levels of heavy metals interfere with gut bacterial balance. In particular, when you have yeast overgrowth—remember Candida from Chapter 2?—if heavy metals are present, it can be very difficult to lower those yeast levels without also addressing the heavy metal toxicity.

An interesting study has brought to light the many toxins we come into contact with daily, often unknowingly. For instance, the artificial sweetener sucralose was found to reduce the amount of beneficial gut microbes, as well as alter the pH and detoxification enzyme levels in an animal model.[41] Sucralose is the nation's bestselling artificial sweetener, used by millions of people, yet it could be contributing to widespread alteration of our good bacteria.

I have covered three common chemical exposures that are known to affect gut balance, but these three examples are probably just the tip of the iceberg. With the sheer number of toxins we encounter every day, the likelihood is great that our digestive balance is being affected. The problem is, toxicity studies are scant and are often based on decades-old models that don't take into account the knowledge we currently hold—especially when it comes to gut bacteria. More research is urgently needed to determine what effects various everyday toxins have on our gut balance.

Remember, the digestive system feeds directly into the liver, the body's main organ of detoxification. Liver function is an important consideration; there's a high prevalence for a condition known as nonalcoholic fatty liver disease (NAFLD), a condition that involves a buildup of fat in the liver. NAFLD is thought to develop as a result of exposure to environmental toxins;[42] it also contributes to the development of obesity and related conditions. In fact, *belly fat is a sign that you may have a fatty liver*. It is estimated that almost 30 percent of adults in the United States have NAFLD. When your digestion functions optimally, your liver has more support in doing its job of detoxification. By achieving a balanced gut on the Skinny Gut Diet, you will give your body the help it needs to effectively deal with toxins.

Obesogens

Not only do environmental toxins knock a person's digestive system off balance, but a wide range of toxins—known as *obesogens*—have been found to trigger weight gain. As toxins that trigger obesity, obesogens do their damage by disrupting hormone function; thus they are known as *endocrine (hormone) disrupting chemicals*. This discovery is relatively recent, but since 2007 the list of toxins that potentially increase weight gain has steadily grown. It includes phthalates, bisphenol A (BPA), flame retardants, perfluorooctanoic acid (PFOA) used in Teflon, polyvinyl chloride (PVC), the pesticide atrazine, DDT, tributyltin, and even triclosan, the additive found in antibacterial soap. These chemicals are in the following items:

- Cash register receipts
- Hand sanitizers
- Nonstick pans
- Plastic bottles with no. 3 and no. 7 recycling symbols
- Shower curtains
- Personal care products

- Air fresheners
- Nail polish
- Sunscreen
- Pajamas
- Tap water

Scientists have found that exposure to obesogens increases fat accumulation not only in individuals exposed to the chemical but also in subsequent generations who did not even come into contact with them. That means that your grandmother's DDT exposure could be the cause of your extra 30 pounds. Now, that's a scary thought.

Could it be that one mechanism by which obesogens lead to weight gain and fat accumulation is through the alteration of our gut microbes? Although the science is still in its infancy, I believe that researchers will indeed find a link between increasing exposure to toxins and gut balance, and that they will find this alteration also leads to weight gain. Reducing our exposure to toxins is important for everyone; what we do know about the effects of these substances on our health is minimal, yet the picture is looking bleak. Fortunately, we can do something about it.

What Can You Do About Toxins?

No one can live in a bubble, free of toxins. Let's be realistic. But we must somehow address the cruel reality that we all carry more than 200 chemical pollutants, pesticides, and toxic metals in our bodies.[43] When your weight loss begins to falter, it's time to consider those other variables that aren't so obvious. I have devised a simple two-step program to help you reduce your exposure to toxins.

Step 1: Minimize the number of toxins in your environment:

- Eat organic foods when possible (or at least eat the Environmental Working Group's Dirty Dozen fruits and vegetables in organic form—see Resources, page 258, for the complete list).

- Use natural cleaners.
- Install water and air filters.

Step 2: Remove the toxins from your body.

- Detoxify and cleanse.
- Take saunas.
- Regularly use herbal cleansing programs and supplements.
- Strongly consider colon hydrotherapy.

See Resources, page 259, for more information about this detoxification program and the supplements you can take to support your body's detoxification.

As our world becomes ever more polluted, our bodies find it harder and harder to cope with the toxins being let loose in the environment. The human body evolved in a natural setting and was designed to cope with common environmental challenges. But, with the help of cleansing herbs and a supportive diet, you can be better prepared to deal with the unique toxic challenges of modern life.

CHAPTER 3 SUMMARY

Gut balance
- ➤ Gut bacterial balance is established early in life and is affected by mode of birth, diet, and antibiotic use during infancy.

Gut imbalance is induced by a number of factors:
- ➤ The environment in which we are raised
- ➤ Antibiotic use
- ➤ Stress
- ➤ Age
- ➤ Use of acid-blocking medications
- ➤ Toxins

Antibiotic resistance

- Antibiotic resistance, triggered by the overuse of antibiotics, is the ability of bacteria to survive in the presence of antibiotics.
- Antibiotic resistance is increasing and is linked to infections that kill over 23,000 people every year.

Everyday toxins linked to obesity

- Obesogens are toxins that trigger obesity via the disruption of hormone function.

What can you do about toxins?

- Minimize toxins in your environment.
- Remove toxins from your body.

Chapter 4

THE PROPER CARE AND FEEDING OF YOUR OWN GUT BACTERIA

There are two probiotic bacteria that are particularly important to human health because they are found in a balanced digestive tract:

- *Bifidobacterium*
- *Lactobacillus*

Bifido and Lacto

I refer to Lactobacilli and Bifidobacteria sometimes as "Lacto" and "Bifido," and sometimes as simply as "the Ls" and "the Bs." Lactobacilli are the most prevalent probiotics in the small (little) intestine, and Bifidobacteria are most prevalent in the colon (big) intestine. The Ls and the Bs are the bacteria that you want more of in your digestive tract. The Skinny Gut Diet will help you get more Ls and Bs.

As you've learned, Bifidobacteria are acquired during natural birth, breast-feeding, and from a diet high in prebiotics. High amounts of Bifidobacteria are associated with less fat, healthier blood sugar levels, and lower digestive toxin levels—all indications of a protective effect against obesity. On the other hand, low levels of Bifidobacteria have been linked with the development of obesity and diabetes.[1] *The more Bifidobacteria you have in your gut, the less likely you are to store fat and gain weight.*

Lactobacillus bacteria are also well known for their health benefits. Lactobacilli are most prevalent in the small intestine, where they produce compounds—such as lactic acid and hydrogen peroxide—that promote a healthy pH level in the digestive tract, inhibiting the growth of harmful bacteria. Lactobacilli are found in foods such as:

- Fermented vegetables
- Kefir
- Certain yogurts
- Other dairy products

There are two ways to restore the balance of your beneficial bacteria, each working in conjunction with the other:

1. Take probiotics that include *Lactobacillus* and *Bifidobacterium,* and take a soluble fiber supplement to help feed the good gut bacteria.
2. Eat a diet high in fiber to help feed the good gut bacteria, and eat plenty of fermented foods that naturally contain good bacteria.

Lactobacillus can also be replenished by taking a probiotic supplement. The use of certain strains of *Lactobacillus* for weight loss is currently being investigated. In a study by researchers in Japan, overweight individuals with excess belly fat were given either fermented milk containing the probiotic *Lactobacillus gasseri* or fermented milk without the added probiotic once daily for twelve weeks.[2] The group drinking the fermented milk with probiotic lost weight, belly fat, and inches off the hips and waist, when compared to the group who drank the fermented milk without added probiotics. The participants did not change their diet or exercise habits; they simply added the *Lactobacillus* probiotic to their milk.

In another study, 159 pregnant women received either a probiotic (*Lactobacillus rhamnosus*) or a placebo from four weeks prior to delivery through six months after delivery.[3] The probiotics were found to reduce excessive weight gain in the first years of life of the infants born to these mothers. Another study in pregnant women found that the probiotics *Lactobacillus rhamnosus* and *Bifidobacterium lactis*, when taken daily from the first trimester through the end of exclusive breast-feeding, helped improve blood sugar control and insulin levels when compared to the placebo.[4]

What About Yogurt?

Could yogurt work in a similar way as probiotics? After all, yogurt is a fermented food, so it should contain these beneficial bacteria, right? Not so fast. I want to clear up some misconceptions about store-bought yogurt. First, not all yogurts contain live probiotic bacteria. In fact, all the yogurt sold in the United States must undergo pasteurization, which heats the milk to kill off potentially pathogenic bacteria. In the process, the good bacteria are also killed. The only yogurt that actually contains probiotic bacteria are the ones that are labeled "contains live cultures." These are yogurts to which live cultures have been added after the pasteurization process, so the end product will still contain probiotic bacteria. The amount of probiotic bacteria, however, is variable owing to the perishable nature of yogurt. The bacteria are continually reproducing inside the yogurt, so the culture count fluctuates, which is why you don't see yogurts touting a specific culture count.

Aside from the fact that your commercial yogurt may not contain *any* beneficial bacteria, the sugar content of most yogurts is very high. All but plain yogurts have added sugars or fruit concentrates that make them not the healthy choice we are led to believe. Next time you are in the grocery store, check out the sugar content of your favorite yogurt. You will be shocked, as I was. While you're there, see if your favorite yogurt brand is labeled "contains live cultures." If so, your best bet is to buy the plain version.

In another study done by Jeffrey Gordon's lab, scientists found that yogurt with live cultures did not change the gut microbiomes of twin individuals who ate it twice a day for four weeks.[5] Gordon explained, "We were only giving several billion bacterial cells in total to the twins, who harbor tens of trillions of gut microbes in their intestines." In short, yogurt does not pack a potent punch when it comes to probiotic activity. If you like plain yogurt, certainly keep eating it, but you will want to also eat living foods and take probiotic and prebiotic supplements to ensure you are replenishing your gut with enough beneficial bacteria.

It pays to have the right bacteria in your gut. Fortunately, you can increase the Bifidobacteria and Lactobacilli probiotics in your gut by eating the right foods and taking the right supplements. My Skinny Gut Diet will show you how.

Prebiotics

Beneficial bacteria thrive on certain soluble fibers known as *pre*biotics because they act as food for the *pro*biotics—the beneficial bacteria in your gut. A diet that includes prebiotic fibers will promote the growth of Bifidobacteria in the digestive tract. The hallmark of a healthy gut diet, prebiotics are found in such common foods as:

- Jerusalem artichoke
- Dandelion greens
- Garlic
- Leeks
- Onions
- Asparagus

The function of prebiotics was first recognized in 1995, when researchers observed that certain fibers beneficially modified the composition of gut bacteria once they were fermented in the gut.[6] Prebiotic fibers are those soluble fibers that support the growth of beneficial gut bacteria, most notably *Bifidobacterium* and, to some extent, *Lactobacillus*. One type of prebiotic fiber, known as *inulin*, is found in the foods I listed above: asparagus, leek, onion, garlic, Jerusalem artichokes, and dandelion greens. Another way to get these beneficial fibers is by taking a prebiotic supplement, which is what has been used in clinical studies that have looked at the effects of prebiotics on weight loss and appetite. Prebiotic supplements are a form of fiber supplement—specifically, a soluble fiber—that has been shown to support the growth of beneficial bacteria.

I will warn you, though, that certain prebiotic supplements can give you a lot of gas. Inulin and fructooligosaccharides (FOS), which are derived from inulin, are gas-forming prebiotics when taken in supplement form. When looking for a prebiotic supplement, you want to ones that have soluble fibers like acacia and non-genetically modified (non-GMO) corn fiber. Find a soluble fiber that mixes clear into a beverage for an easy way to get your prebiotic fiber boost. Read the label to make sure you are getting the right one.

"Life is great these days. I make good food choices and my body loves me for it. Having the energy to live my life fully and know that my gut is balanced and life is good is the biggest reward of the Skinny Gut Diet." —Polly

In a study of overweight and obese individuals, those who took a prebiotic twice daily experienced better appetite satisfaction after breakfast and dinner, along with a reduction in hunger and food intake following dinner, when compared to those who only took the placebo.[7] And in a follow-up to this study, individuals who took a prebiotic twice daily experienced reduced hunger along with increases in two proteins (glucagon-like peptide 1 and peptide YY) that are excreted in the intestines in response to food, increasing feelings of fullness and decreased appetite.[8] Accompanying this decrease in hunger was an increase in the fermentation activity by gut bacteria, which suggests the gut bacteria are responsible for the appetite effects.

By simply feeding your gut bacteria with prebiotic fibers, you can improve your gut balance and reduce your appetite. Unfortunately, it's

SKINNY GUT SUCCESS STORY: CHARLIE M.

Charlie is a 36-year-old financial adviser with a high-stress job that re-quires long hours and excellent focus. Fortunately, Charlie is an over-all healthy guy. When he began the Skinny Gut Diet, he didn't notice any obvious signs of digestive distress.

Like so many adults, as Charlie's job and home responsibilities in-creased over time, his exercise level decreased—and his weight went up. His desire was to be 20 pounds lighter for his upcoming wedding. Charlie is a food-conscious individual, so when he learned the princi-ples of the Skinny Gut Diet, it made sense to him.

Eating at regular intervals has been helpful in regulating Charlie's food intake at his workplace. He preplans his lunches and makes sure he has protein snacks and even dinner options always available. This commitment added to Charlie's sharpness of mind and disciplined at-titude in all areas of his life. And his weight steadily reduced.

Interestingly, lab testing revealed Charlie as the "buggiest" guy in our client population—his gut bacteria were very much out of bal-ance. His test showed that he was positive for opportunistic bacteria, pathogenic *H. pylori,* and the highest measurable reading of yeast. Add to that, his adiposity index showed that he had the classic "obese gut type"—high Firmicutes (Fat bacteria) and low Bacteroidetes (Be Skinny bacteria). And yet Charlie didn't notice any digestive discom-fort.

This is the perfect example of something I have witnessed count-less times. So often our guts can be far out of balance without any obvious digestive symptoms. It's critical that you realize that weight gain is an indication that your gut is out of balance, which is the start-ing point for inflammation and chronic disease. Where does this trou-ble come from? Excess sugar and starchy carbohydrates in the diet feed the bad bacteria that can ultimately result in weight loss and poor health.

```
ADIPOSITY INDEX
         CHARLIE

BEFORE:                            Expected
                                    Value

  Firmicutes %  76  [======◆==]    < = 80%
  Bacteroidetes %  24  [==◆======]  > = 20%


AFTER:                             Expected
                                    Value

  Firmicutes %  56  [====◆====]    < = 80%
  Bacteroidetes %  44  [===◆=====]  > = 20%
```

"I generally feel thinner and look thinner, but I actually feel as though I am lighter—I never feel heavy like I used to after eating a big meal." —Charlie

After just six weeks on the Skinny Gut Diet, the opportunistic bacteria and yeast had diminished and Charlie's "obese gut type" had transformed into a "lean gut type." By the end of three months, Charlie had lost 21 pounds. He feels great, looks great, and now has a new appreciation for eating healthy. He told me that he wasn't able to exercise as much as he would have liked, but he didn't feel the negative effects of not exercising because of how well he was eating.

Charlie	Weight	Waistline Inches	Body Fat %
Before	188	40"	26.9%
After	167	34¾"	19.5%
Lost	21 lb	5¼"	7.4%

not easy to get enough fiber through diet alone. A fiber supplement is a simple and effective way to reach your daily fiber goal and improve your gut balance. Likewise, the ten overweight individuals on my successful Skinny Gut Diet program (described earlier) took a daily fiber supplement. See Resources, page 255, for my recommended products.

CHAPTER 4 SUMMARY

The Impressive Performance of Probiotics and Prebiotics
➤ There are two probiotic bacteria that are particularly important to human health because they are found in a balanced digestive tract:

Bifidobacterium
Lactobacillus

➤ Prebiotics are soluble fibers that act as food for probiotics. Prebiotics are found in such foods as chicory root, Jerusalem artichoke, dandelion greens, garlic, leek, onion, and asparagus.
➤ Probiotics and prebiotics help to restore gut balance by increasing the beneficial bacteria and decreasing the harmful bacteria.

What About Yogurt?
➤ Aside from the fact that your yogurt may not contain *any* beneficial bacteria, the sugar content of most store-bought yogurt is very high. Be sure to read your label.

Chapter 5

YOUR GUT CONNECTION TO OBESITY AND OTHER COMMON CONDITIONS

The seemingly modest digestive tract, while busy breaking down food into small, usable nutrients, also serves an equally important role of housing up to 80 percent of the body's immune system.[1] That's right—the majority of your immune system is in your gut. When you think of immune health, you probably envision being stuffed up with a cold or run down with the flu. Digestion is likely the last thing that comes to mind when you think of immune health, but nothing could be further from the truth. The body's largest accumulation of immune cells is situated in and around the intestinal tract, and they are intricately dependent on digestive health.

Your gut microbes educate your immune system so that it knows how to appropriately respond. If your gut microbes are made up of a diverse balance of the right kind of bacteria, your bacteria will school your immune system so that it makes peace with the food you eat, the occasional pathogens you harbor, and the toxins you ingest. If the composition of your gut microbes is out of balance, on the other hand, the microbes do not properly educate your immune system and it will either fight everything it encounters—foods, pathogens, toxins, and even your own tissues—or not fight strongly enough and the pathogens win.

Silent Inflammation

When you think of inflammation, you probably think of joint pain, cuts, or something that hurts. But inflammation cannot always be felt. When your immune system fights harmless substances or low-level pathogens, it produces silent inflammation, a chronic, low-grade inflammation that you can't see or feel, but that simmers in your gut and damages the intestinal lining. Destruction to the intestinal lining increases its permeability, a condition known as leaky gut, which was explained earlier. When the intestinal lining is damaged, the immune system is presented with an increase in bacteria, toxins, and even undigested food particles, which trigger yet more inflammation that now enters the circulation and can affect many different areas of the body. Silent inflammation is the thread that connects gut imbalance to obesity, as well as a wide range of chronic health conditions.

Gut imbalance → Silent inflammation → Obesity

The ability of the gut microbes to educate the immune system is crucial to health because the body's immune response is tied to most, if not all, chronic health conditions. An imbalanced immune response involves either too little response, as found in people who seem to catch every bug that goes around, or too much response, as is seen in the inflammation-driven chronic diseases such as diabetes, heart disease, and allergies that have reached epidemic proportions in our modern (gut-imbalanced) world. However, a balanced gut bacterial composition establishes a balanced immune response, and a balanced immune response means the immune system is responding as it should. In a word, immune balance means inflammation balance. There is no chronic, silent inflammation when the immune system is balanced.

Obesity is usually characterized by silent inflammation, and it is accompanied by the development of insulin resistance, the condition whereby insulin (the hormone that regulates blood sugar) does not function properly, eventually resulting in high blood sugar.[2] The origin of the silent inflammation found in people with obesity was not entirely understood until recently. As it turns out, gut imbalance is a major source of the inflammation that drives obesity. When you balance your gut, you will quell the silent inflammation at its source, and you will help to reverse the disease process that leads to obesity. The Skinny Gut Diet gives you the tools to do so.

DIGESTIVE CONDITIONS

While gut imbalance can lead to digestive conditions, as well as to issues outside the digestive tract, digestive conditions themselves can lead to gut imbalance. It's a two-way road. Digestive conditions lead to gut imbalance and gut imbalance leads to digestive conditions. The following are just a few of the most common digestive states that can throw off gut balance. Getting these conditions under control is imperative. Fortunately, the Skinny Gut Diet will help you address them.

Constipation

Constipation is defined as infrequent or incomplete bowel movements, often characterized by stools that are hard, dry, and difficult to pass owing to slow transit time through the gastrointestinal tract. Gut transit time is the amount of time that elapses between ingestion of food and its excretion in the form of stool.

In conventional medical circles, it is considered normal to have a bowel movement as infrequently as three times a week.[3] In contrast, integrative health practitioners consider the normal range of bowel movements to be one to three per day. A daily bowel movement may still be considered constipation if the amount of feces eliminated is small or very hard. A daily bowel movement that is well formed and about one and a half feet long is considered normal by natural health practitioners. This may be broken up into two or three bowel movements per day or, sometimes, just one. I have consulted with so many people over the years who consider having only one bowel movement weekly is normal. Some people are so constipated that they have only one bowel movement *per month*. Can you imagine what is happening on the inside at that point? It's a scary thought.

When you are constipated, digestive contents remain in the intestines for longer periods of time, putrefying as the intestinal bacteria ferment what's left of the food you ate. The longer food sits in the colon, the more appealing it is for the harmful bacteria that produce toxic compounds and gases to gain an upper hand over the beneficial bacteria, which cannot as easily survive in the toxic environment of the constipated gut.[4]

> **"Before the Skinny Gut Diet, laxatives were one of my basic food groups. I was constipated during my entire adult life, so I did what I knew best: take a laxative. I had no idea what I was doing internally to my digestive system. During the program, I learned to replace laxatives with green vegetables and juices, probiotics, fiber, and a healthy diet. I am consistent now with daily movements."**
> **—Cynthia**

One of the main causes of constipation is a lack of dietary fiber. An ideal daily diet should contain 35 grams of fiber, which helps promote bowel regularity by bulking up the stool and feeding the beneficial gut bacteria (remember, fiber is a prebiotic). Unfortunately, the Standard American Diet (SAD) contains less than half of our daily fiber needs. And even with a healthy diet high in nonstarchy vegetables and low-sugar fruits, it can be difficult to consume 35 grams of fiber daily. That's why I recommend taking a daily fiber supplement in addition to eating a healthy diet. That way you can be sure you are getting all your daily fiber. See Chapter 11 for more about fiber's crucial role in maintaining a healthy gut.

Other causes of constipation include:

- Standard American Diet
- Certain medications (antidepressants, tranquilizers, certain painkillers, and certain blood pressure and heart medications)
- Lack of exercise
- Major life changes
- Travel
- Pregnancy
- Excessive use of laxatives or enemas
- Ignoring the urge to defecate
- Surgery (such as hysterectomy or back surgery that may result in severance of nerves in the bowel)
- Dehydration
- Extreme stress or depression
- Magnesium deficiency
- Certain nutrient deficiencies
- Prolonged bed rest
- Lack of sleep
- Advanced age
- Spinal cord injury
- Insufficient levels of digestive enzymes

The Skinny Gut Diet will help you achieve bowel regularity and gut balance. The high-fiber, high-nutrient diet, along with digestive support supplements, will keep your digestion moving at a healthy rate so that constipation is no longer a problem.

Irritable Bowel Syndrome

Irritable bowel syndrome (IBS) is usually identified by a group of symptoms. This condition is often determined more by what it is not than by what it is. IBS is characterized by the predominant symptoms of abdominal pain and altered bowel habits (constipation and/or diarrhea). It is a chronic condition that can last years or even a lifetime,

SKINNY GUT SUCCESS STORY: CYNTHIA B.

When Cynthia joined our Skinny Gut group, I had no idea that she might have been voted Least Likely to Succeed. Cynthia, at age 58, was a bona fide junk-food junkie. She told me that she had never purchased 90 percent of the foods on the Skinny Gut Diet. She didn't even know what many of them were.

After decades of frustration at her previous corporate job, Cynthia had learned to turn to food as her best friend. Let me rephrase that, as I wouldn't consider much of what Cynthia ate as food. Her "friend" was sugar in all forms. Whether she ate pizza, candy, cookies, potato chips, or drive-through fast food, there were chemicals and carbs in almost every mouthful.

As she was chronically constipated, it wasn't unusual for Cynthia to go seven days without a bowel movement. Frustrated with feeling so stopped up, she took to carrying around a bottle of water with Miralax in it for relief. In addition, Cynthia frequently experienced sciatic back pain and constantly had pain in her joints. No wonder she felt irritable, awkward, and exhausted. She told me that the depression following her pain would land her in bed with a quart of ice cream for comfort.

Today, Cynthia regularly makes blended green drinks to "get the green stuff in." She is still not a big fan of veggies, but she knows she needs them. And she learned to like fermented foods. She has left behind the cakes, cookies, and candies, finding substitutes to fill that void without destroying her health.

but with proper diet and supplements, IBS can be well controlled and even alleviated.

Several digestive conditions have similar symptoms as IBS, including malabsorption (impairment in the absorption of nutrients), in-

"When I began the Skinny Gut Diet, I didn't know what I was signing up for. I fought and kicked my way through it, and suddenly I am 20 pounds lighter. And my gut is happy. I would not say it is a diet, but it certainly helped me to lose weight, and I am not in pain anymore. And yes—I am eating those leafy greens."
—Cynthia

On the Skinny Gut Diet, Cynthia now experiences daily bowel movements and has found that her pains are gone—even the sciatica. (Incidentally, sciatica often shows up along with the inflammation of constipation.) She goes on long walks with ease, and her mind is clearer than it has been in years. She swears she is never going back. She has dropped 20 pounds and is well on her way toward reaching her 30-pound weight-loss goal. She has her slinky dress all picked out for the next holiday season.

That's not all. Cynthia's 79-year-old mother was visiting her while she was on the Skinny Gut Diet, and she followed Cynthia's example by partially shifting her diet as well. She lost 14 pounds. Cynthia is thrilled that her mother's weight is moving in a heart-healthy direction, and she knows her mother's doctor will be, too.

Cynthia	Weight	Waistline Inches	Body Fat %
Before	185	41¾"	42.0%
After	165	34¼"	36.7%
Lost	20 lbs	7½"	5.3%

flammatory bowel disease (such as ulcerative colitis and Crohn's disease), celiac disease, lactose intolerance, Candida overgrowth, and intestinal parasites, all of which are associated with gut bacterial imbalance as either a contributing factor or a result of the

SKINNY GUT SUCCESS STORY: SANDI M.

Sandi is a very pleasant and energetic 61-year-old woman. Early in the Skinny Gut Diet program she said that she doubted she would ever get back into the clothes she had been storing for years in vacuum packs in the back of her closet. Her weight had slowly crept up over the years, leaving her with 25 extra pounds that she had been carrying for the last three years. With regard to her weight, Sandi vacillated between frustration and resignation.

As a child, Sandi had received many rounds of antibiotics for earaches and tonsillitis. Looking back, she realizes that she had been battling Candida and yeast issues for most of her adult life, which showed up as sinus problems, at times vaginitis, and of course, weight gain.

Fortunately for Sandi, it wasn't that she ate large portions of food daily or that she made poor food choices overall. Digestive health was not a new concept to her. In fact, she had been taking digestive support supplements for years. What the test did uncover, however, was substantial yeast overgrowth.

On the Skinny Gut Diet, Sandi eliminated gluten products and decreased her carbohydrate intake, which stopped feeding her yeast. As she learned to count teaspoons of sugar, after all those years her weight finally began to reduce steadily. In follow-up testing, Sandi no longer showed evidence of yeast overgrowth. Carbs had admittedly been her downfall.

Sandi dropped 16 pounds over three months and now fits into many of the smaller clothes she had packed away in her closet. In fact—she

condition—or both. (It's another vicious cycle.) IBS affects up to one in five adults, yet most of them have not been diagnosed.[5] Women are affected twice as often as men, and both are usually affected before the age of 45.

went from a size 16 to a size 10. She looks forward to donating the larger clothes—certain now that she won't need them anymore. Sandi calls it healthy weight loss, especially since weight loss during midlife and beyond can be a challenge. It's a skinny gut for life.

> **"I have noticed that I feel so great! I have more energy, and I see myself lose inches as my clothes are getting baggier. It is a wonderful experience!"** —Sandi

Sandi has also enjoyed an unexpected benefit. She had been previously diagnosed with a heart arrhythmia by her cardiologist and takes medication to lessen the intensity and frequency of the palpitations. At the beginning of the Skinny Gut Diet program her palpitations were frequent. Interestingly, after a month on the Skinny Gut Diet, Sandi realized that the palpitations were almost gone. She looks forward to sharing this finding with her doctor very soon. What a terrific added perk for her.

Sandi	Weight	Waistline Inches	Body Fat %
Before	171	37½″	44.3%
After	155	33″	38.9%
Lost	16 lbs	4½″	5.4%

The bacterial imbalance that occurs with IBS must be addressed in order to find relief from its symptoms and achieve lasting weight loss. If you are suffering from IBS, the Skinny Gut Diet will help you rebalance your gut and get IBS under control.

Candida (Yeast) Overgrowth

The presence of *Candida albicans*—a benign, sugar-fermenting yeast—on the skin and in the mouth, on the genitals, and especially in the intestinal tract is a normal occurrence when numbers of the yeast are low. As was discussed in Chapter 2, in small amounts this microbe is part of the intestinal ecology in most people, and when kept in balance with other microorganisms, it does not cause harm. But when Candida grows out of control, no longer being kept in check by the beneficial microbes in the gut, a yeast imbalance results. Candida overgrowth in the gut releases toxic waste products when it proliferates, causing an array of symptoms that range from chronic fatigue, brain fog, and headache to sugar cravings, gas, bloating, and yeast infections.

Although the most common, Candida is not the only yeast organism that grows out of control. Yeast overgrowth may involve yeasts other than Candida as well. But no matter the source, yeast overgrowth can be a hindrance to successful weight loss and must be addressed if you want to shed weight. If you think you may have yeast overgrowth, you can be tested for it by using a stool test from an integrative medical lab. (See Resources, page 257, for recommended labs.) The main cause of Candida overgrowth is antibiotic use. Candida is a yeast, not a bacteria, and antibiotics only kill bacteria. So yeasts have the opportunity to take the upper hand after the antibiotics have wiped out all the beneficial bacteria that normally keep the yeast growth in check.

> Fully 100 percent of the participants in my Skinny Gut Diet program started off with elevated levels of yeast in their digestive tracts. Addressing yeast overgrowth is a vital part of rebalancing the gut.

You may remember that Candida feeds on sugar, which helps explain the sugar and carbohydrate cravings common in people with yeast overgrowth. Eliminating sugar and starchy carbohydrates is crucial for getting that Candida overgrowth under control. The Skinny Gut Diet is naturally low in sugar to help starve the bad microbes—Candida in particular—and high in fiber to help feed the beneficial bacteria. By eating the right foods and taking the right supplements, you can create a friendly environment that supports the growth of beneficial bacteria while keeping the harmful microbes at bay. In more complicated cases, diet may not be enough to address yeast overgrowth. In that case, look for a thirty-day Candida cleanse supplement program that contains antifungal herbs that target yeast. (See Resources, page 255, for my product recommendations.)

Acid Reflux and Heartburn

Heartburn, also known as acid reflux or acid indigestion, is a condition in which partially digested food from the stomach, along with stomach acid and enzymes, backs up into the esophagus. The process is known as reflux. When it creates a burning sensation that then radiates upward, it is known as heartburn. The term *heartburn* is used to describe an individual event, but the medical term for chronic (frequent) heartburn is *gastroesophageal reflux disease* (GERD). Heartburn is considered GERD when it occurs two or more times per week.

Stomach acid, or hydrochloric acid (HCl), has a low pH, meaning that it is very acidic. Even if it's present in low amounts, HCl can cause damage when it comes into contact with the delicate lining of the esophagus. This mucous lining, or mucosa, of the esophagus, unlike the lining of the stomach, is not designed to withstand the caustic effects of acid and stomach contents.

There are a number of dietary and lifestyle factors that may contribute to esophageal irritation. These include:

- Overeating
- Eating too rapidly
- Inadequate chewing

- Overweight/obesity
- Lying down after eating
- Tight-fitting clothing that constricts the abdomen
- Stress (and eating when upset)
- Alcoholic beverages
- Smoking
- Chocolate and peppermint
- Spicy foods
- Tomato- and citrus-based foods
- Fried foods
- Sugar
- Coffee, tea, and other caffeine-containing beverages
- Certain medications (NSAIDs like aspirin, ibuprofen, and naproxen; the antibiotic tetracycline; the antiarrhythmic drug quinidine; potassium chloride; and iron salts)
- Food allergies and sensitivities (especially to wheat and dairy)
- Gallbladder problems
- Hiatal hernia
- Enzyme deficiencies

Unfortunately, instead of getting to the root cause of the acid reflux, most people are put on proton pump inhibitors (PPIs) to shut down the production of stomach acid. Short-term use of PPIs can be helpful to relieve symptoms for the initial phase of healing, but long-term use of these medications is linked to many negative health effects. Acid-blocking medication was originally developed for short-term treatment of gut irritation. But today, PPIs are the third-highest-selling drug on the market and many people remain on them for many years. The side effects of long-term PPI use include:

- Increased risk of *Clostridium difficile* (C. diff) infection[6]
- Candida overgrowth in the esophagus[7]

- Osteoporosis-related bone fractures[8]
- Pneumonia[9]
- Vitamin B12 deficiency[10]

If you have GERD and are on acid-blocking medication over the long term, find an integrative medical doctor (see Resources, page 257) who can work with you to carefully wean you off these medications with the proper dietary changes and digestive enzymes. For guidance, ask your doctor if you can slowly give up these drugs using my Acid Blocker Recovery protocol (in the Resources, page 262). I have designed the Skinny Gut Diet to support digestive health. You may find on your own, as participants of my Skinny Gut Diet program did, that this diet resolves your heartburn symptoms.

Diarrhea

Diarrhea is the frequent passage of watery stools. Diarrhea may be either acute or chronic. Acute diarrhea takes the form of an isolated incident caused by a temporary problem—usually an infection that lasts three to seven days. Chronic diarrhea, though, is much more complex with a multitude of causes, and it can last for months or even years. Basically, the condition stems from intestinal irritation or increased motility (muscular action) in the intestinal tract that can be brought on by a variety or causes, including:

- Incomplete digestion of food
- Use of certain medications (especially antibiotics and NSAIDs) that damage the gut lining
- Food allergies or sensitivities
- Excessive alcohol consumption
- Regular or excessive intake of caffeine
- Overuse of sugar and sweeteners
- Infections (bacterial, yeast, or parasitic)

- Emotional stress
- Bowel diseases
- Radiation or chemotherapy
- Nutrient deficiencies
- Celiac disease or gluten sensitivity
- Use of magnesium-containing antacids
- Long-distance running
- Pancreatic insufficiency

SKINNY GUT DIET SUCCESS: DAVE M.

Dave is truly a man on a mission. He tells me that he had heard me state the often-asked question, "Are you sick and tired of being sick and tired?" and it took up residence in his soul. When he started the Skinny Gut Diet he was sick and tired, and really committed to doing something about it.

In 1991, when Dave, 6 feet tall, left the service, he weighed 189 pounds. Over the years he steadily gained weight, at one point tipping the scale at 315 pounds. It was his highest weight and a low point in his life. For the last few years, through his attempts at calorie restriction and better food choices—all motivated by frightening lab test results delivered by his doctor at the VA hospital—he had lowered his weight to just below 300. Dave's health showed the effects of the Standard American Diet. Like so many his age, Dave found himself taking cholesterol-lowering prescriptions, blood thinners, and blood pressure medications. Yet even medicated, Dave's blood pressure defied stability and remained high most of the time.

Dave began the Skinny Gut Diet program at 285 pounds. He left gluten and grains behind and began counting his teaspoons of sugar using my unique Teaspoon Tracker calculation. As he embraced the high-quality proteins and enjoyed fermented and natural foods, I'm thrilled to tell you that his blood pressure stabilized dramatically. His diastolic pressure has been under 80 and his systolic rarely reaches 130 (normal adult blood pressure is 120/80).

For people with chronic diarrhea who have ruled out more serious bowel diseases, the Skinny Gut Diet may help you address the root cause of your symptoms. The Skinny Gut Diet removes wheat and gluten from the diet, replenishes your digestive tract with beneficial bacteria, and provides plenty of fiber to help bulk up your stool, all of which may help to clear up chronic diarrhea. If you find that you still have chronic diarrhea on the diet, find an integrative medical doctor (see Resources, page 257) to help you get to the root cause of your condition.

Throughout Dave's adult life, he had experienced loose bowel movements, to the point that he simply considered that to be normal. I am here to tell you that's not normal. As we focused on balancing Dave's gut by replenishing his good bacteria and starving his yeast, along with rebuilding his intestinal lining, Dave's bowel movements began to normalize. Dave now experiences well-formed stools on a daily basis. That one result will have wonderful effects on Dave's ability to absorb nutrients and on his immune function (remember that up to 80 percent of the immune system resides in the gut). In addition, Dave's Fat bacteria decreased and his Be Skinny bacteria increased.

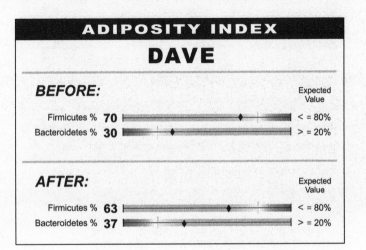

ADIPOSITY INDEX

DAVE

BEFORE:

		Expected Value
Firmicutes % **70**		< = 80%
Bacteroidetes % **30**		> = 20%

AFTER:

		Expected Value
Firmicutes % **63**		< = 80%
Bacteroidetes % **37**		> = 20%

"I first thought this was going to be a useless uphill battle,
but after a short while I realized that the lifestyle change wasn't
the ordeal that I made it out to be in the beginning.
I am feeling better than I have ever felt before." —Dave

Dave lost 39 pounds in the first three months on the Skinny Gut Diet program and he continues to follow the diet and to lose weight. He is a new and healthy man. It will be great to see what weight his body normalizes at with his newly balanced gut. I expect that over time he will be able to lower or even come off of his medications while working closely with his doctor. Dave's energy is great and his enthusiasm is contagious. No more "sick and tired" for Dave. He will tell you that he has truly embraced the Skinny Gut Diet program for life.

Dave	Weight	Waistline Inches	Body Fat %
Before	285	50"	42.9%
After	246	41½"	37.0%
Lost	39 lbs	8½"	5.9%

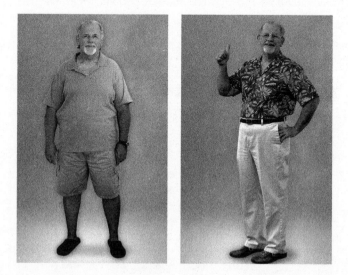

Before and After

CHAPTER 5 SUMMARY

Silent Inflammation

➤ Silent inflammation is a chronic, low-grade inflammation that you can't see or feel. When you balance your gut, you will quell the silent inflammation and help to reverse the disease process that leads to obesity.

Digestive Conditions

➤ **Constipation:** When you are constipated, digestive contents remain in the intestines for longer periods of time, putrefying as intestinal bacteria ferment what's left of the food you ate. The longer food sits in the colon, the more appealing it is for harmful bacteria that produce toxic compounds and gases as they gain an upper hand over the beneficial bacteria that cannot as easily survive in the toxic environment of the constipated gut.

➤ **Irritable bowel syndrome:** The bacterial imbalance that occurs with IBS must be addressed in order to find relief from symptoms and to achieve lasting weight loss.

➤ **Candida overgrowth:** Candida overgrowth in the gut—which is a form of gut imbalance—releases toxic waste products when it proliferates, causing an array of symptoms that range from chronic fatigue, brain fog, and headache to sugar cravings, gas, bloating, and yeast infections.

➤ **Acid reflux:** Heartburn, also known as acid reflux or acid indigestion, is a condition in which partially digested food from the stomach, along with stomach acid and enzymes, backs up into the esophagus.

➤ **Diarrhea:** Diarrhea is the frequent passage of watery stools. Basically, the condition stems from intestinal irritation or increased motility (muscular action) in the intestinal tract that can be brought on by a variety or causes.

Chapter 6

THE GUT-BRAIN CONNECTION

Not only does digestive imbalance lead to obesity, but it also contributes to the development of conditions that occur alongside obesity. The silent inflammation produced as a result of the wrong balance of microbes in the gut is also found in people with depression and anxiety. Researchers think the silent inflammation is actually *causing* the depression and anxiety symptoms, in many cases. *If you have experienced depression or anxiety, did you ever think it could be caused by your digestion?* This discovery is changing how some researchers and doctors evaluate and treat mood disorders. Replenishing beneficial bacteria in the gut has been shown to reduce symptoms of stress and anxiety, strengthening the evidence that a balanced gut means a balanced mood.[1]

It may seem implausible that your digestive system has anything to do with how your brain functions, but the gut is actually considered to be your second brain, owing to the presence of the enteric nervous system, a branch of the autonomic nervous system that resides in the gut and is responsible for digestive functions. Inside your gut can be found the main neurotransmitters used in the brain. In fact, 95 percent of the body's serotonin, the neurotransmitter responsible for feelings of well-being and happiness, is produced in the intestines.

The gut-brain connection seems obvious when we consider the effects of emotional stress on our digestion. But this connection travels both ways. That is, conditions that involve the brain and mood affect digestive function, and, conversely, digestive conditions affect brain and mood function. Think about it: when you are feeling stressed out or emotionally upset, does your stomach also bother you? You have probably experienced a lack of appetite in a highly stressed situation. Experts have known about the brain's effects on the gut for a long time now. But what they did not realize until relatively recently was the opposite possibility: that digestive dysfunction can actually *cause* mood imbalance. This recently discovered phenomenon is changing how scientists view the gut-brain connection.

The gut-brain connection travels via three main paths: the nervous system, the immune system, and the endocrine, or hormonal, system. All three systems are intricately tied to brain and mood function. Gut imbalance triggers silent inflammation, which is found in people with depression and anxiety, and is thought to play an important role in the development of these mood disorders.[2] Gut inflammation is thought to influence the three gut-brain pathways, traveling to the brain. That means that what happens in your gut can affect your mind. Could the fact that many people do not respond to mood-regulating drugs have anything to do with an underlying gut imbalance? If so, then balancing the gut would help to improve their symptoms.

Gut Balance and Your Mood

Indeed, researchers have been investigating the use of probiotics in people with mood symptoms. Probiotic intake has been found to reduce anxiety, decrease stress response, and improve mood in people with irritable bowel syndrome (IBS) and chronic fatigue syndrome. Probiotics have also been found to help reduce symptoms of anxiety and the stress hormone cortisol.[3] In these people, simply balancing the gut with probiotics helped improve mood and reduce stress. Reducing inflammation in the gut can help. Studies like these are shaking up the scientific community in a big way.

GUT SCIENCE WITH DR. LEONARD SMITH

Probiotics for the Mind—Psychobiotics

Use of probiotics to benefit mood is a recent advancement in the scientific literature, first proposed in 2005 when researchers suggested its use as an adjuvant (add-on) treatment to standard care for major depressive disorder.[4] In 2013, scientists defined *psychobiotic* as "a live organism that, when ingested in adequate amounts, produces a health benefit in patients suffering from psychiatric illness," recommending them as a novel class of psychotropic (mind-altering) treatment.[5] Probiotics have been found to act as delivery vehicles for neuroactive compounds (compounds that stimulate the nervous system), and certain probiotic strains actually secrete these neuroactive compounds.[6]

In animal models, the probiotic *Bifidobacterium infantis* was found to increase the serotonin precursor tryptophan.[7] Serotonin is the feel-good hormone, and many antidepressant medications work by increasing its availability in the body. Might probiotics one day fill the role of antidepressant? Time will tell. So far the studies indicate that it's a good possibility. In another animal model, *Bifidobacterium infantis* was found to normalize immune response, reverse negative behavioral effects, and restore norepinephrine (noradrenaline) levels induced by stress. *Lactobacillus rhamnosus* has been found to reduce anxiety and alter expression of GABA (gamma-aminobutyric acid) receptors, in another animal model.[8] GABA is a calming neurotransmitter that has a counterbalancing effect to anxiety.

Researchers have also found that replacing the gut microbes of timid mice with those from mice that exhibit bold, exploratory behavior changed the behavior of the mice from timid to bold.[9] When they replaced the microbes of the bold mice with those from the timid mice, the same thing happened: the bold mice became more timid. The researchers of this study concluded that gut imbalance might contribute to psychiatric disorders in patients with bowel disorders.

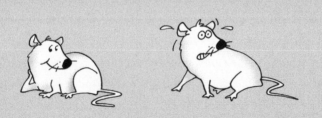

It turns out that intestinal microbes actually help shape the development of the hypothalamic-pituitary-adrenal (HPA) axis. The HPA axis links the hypothalamus and pituitary gland in the brain with the adrenal glands that control stress response. Together, the HPA axis controls many processes in the body, including stress response, digestion, immunity, mood, and metabolism, to name a few. Studies have found that mice raised to be germ free responded in an exaggerated way to mild stress when compared to mice with microbes in their guts.[10] When those microbes were transplanted into the germ-free mice, the exaggerated stress response was partially reversed. When the germ-free mice were repopulated with *Bifidobacterium infantis*, the exaggerated stress response completely normalized.

This shows that gut microbes—Bifidobacteria, in particular— positively affect the body's response to stress. According to scientists, "This study clearly demonstrated that the microbial content of the gut is critical to the development of an appropriate stress response later in life and also that there is a narrow window in early life when colonization must occur to ensure normal development of the HPA axis."[11] The study highlights the importance of establishing gut balance during infancy on mental health later in life.

Human studies have also found benefits from probiotics on mood. In one study, individuals who took a combination of the probiotics *Lactobacillus helveticus* and *Bifidobacterium longum* for thirty days experienced reduced psychological distress and decreased cortisol levels (cortisol is a hormone released under stress), when compared to those who took the placebo. Another human study found that healthy individuals who consumed a probiotic yogurt (yogurt that contains live probiotic bacteria) for three weeks, and who had the lowest mood at the beginning of the study, reported that they were happy rather than depressed after taking the probiotic yogurt. And in a study of patients with chronic fatigue syndrome, those taking *Lactobacillus casei* three times daily for two months experienced an improvement in anxiety when compared to those taking placebo. [12]

And in another study of women who ate a yogurt containing probiotics versus women who ate yogurt without probiotics and women who did not eat any yogurt at all, those women who ate the yogurt with probiotics were found to have areas of the brain activated that control central processing of emotion and sensation when compared to the other women.[13] This study clearly demonstrates that what happens in the gut affects the brain. "Time and time again, we hear from patients that they never felt depressed or anxious until they started experiencing problems with their gut," stated the lead researcher. "Our study shows that the gut-brain connection is a two-way street."

Also interesting to note, similar to antibiotics, antipsychotic medications have been found to alter the gut microbial balance by decreasing the amount of Actinobacteria (of which the beneficial *Bifidobacterium* is a member) and Proteobacteria while increasing the number of Firmicutes (Fat bacteria).[14] Likely not a coincidence that these individuals also gained weight.

As we continue to learn more about how our gut microbes affect mood, it is clear that probiotics—or psychobiotics, as these researchers have termed them—will play an important role in managing or possibly even preventing mood disorders.

If an imbalance of gut bacteria is capable of increasing your waistline and making you more prone to depression and anxiety, you'll want to do everything you can to restore balance that will become the very foundation of your overall health. I wrote this book to show you how to do that. Fortunately, you can balance your gut by eating the right foods and taking the right supplements. Eating living foods and taking probiotics will help to replenish the beneficial probiotic bacteria you may be missing, and eating foods high in fiber and taking additional prebiotic fiber supplements will help feed those beneficial bacteria so that you can achieve and maintain gut balance, and thereby reap the rewards of better mood and mental well-being.

SKINNY GUT SUCCESS STORY: THERESA M.

Theresa is a very attractive 51-year-old woman who has slowly witnessed 30 pounds creep onto her lovely figure over the last twenty years. She told me at the beginning of the Skinny Gut Diet program that she was feeling out of control in her life, mentally foggy, and insecure. She had suffered from constipation her entire life. She also told me that she was nauseous every evening as she went to bed. She even joked about all the money she spent on nausea medication.

A good cook, excellent baker, and devoted grandmother and wife, Theresa prided herself on serving the foods that her family loved—foods that, alas, were not always considered healthy. Fortunately she naturally enjoys green vegetables and salads. In fact, I'm quite sure that is one reason she wasn't heavier.

Theresa's life changed on the Skinny Gut Diet. Her daily nausea disappeared, her constipation was relieved, and her mental fogginess cleared. Her husband even told me that her self-esteem improved. Theresa lost 16 pounds in the first three months on the Skinny Gut Diet without becoming overwhelmed by sugar cravings. She is now learning new ways to create delicious, healthful foods and baked goods using low-carb alternative flours and sweeteners. She now understands that carbs and sugars are the underlying causes for many of the issues that afflict her loved ones.

That's not all. Theresa began with an obese gut type—lots of Fat bacteria and not enough Be Skinny bacteria. But on the Skinny Gut Diet, her gut bacteria reverted back to a lean gut type.

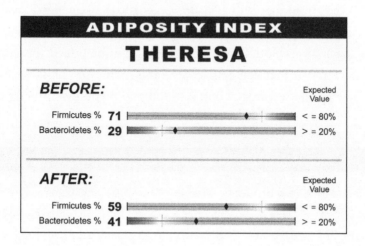

"No more upset stomach or cramping. And the added bonus— I went down a pant size. That's a big accomplishment for me."
—Theresa

I really admire Theresa. Although her husband is thrilled with the new Theresa, commenting enthusiastically on how great she looks, neither he nor her close friends or granddaughter have been willing to accept her new lifestyle. They call her "crazy." Theresa has actually managed to change her life with very little support from home. If lack of support or even resistance at home is a problem you face, know that you are not alone. Many men and women are going through your same struggle and those that come out on the other side will be healthier, skinnier, and more empowered than ever. At that point, the naysayers will no longer have reason to hold you back. They'll see how great you look and feel and will likely change their tune.

Have you ever been called out for stepping outside of what others deem to be normal in order to take a stand and improve yourself? Well, I certainly have. And I am happy to say that my health seems to get better and better. I am stronger and happier than ever—at 60! Sometimes crazy is a good thing to be. Theresa, you have my vigorous applause and continued support.

Theresa	Weight	Waistline Inches	Body Fat %
Before	157	36¼"	40.8%
After	141	30"	34.6%
Lost	16 lbs	6¼"	6.2%

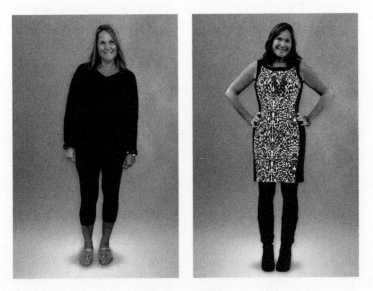

Before and After

CHAPTER 6 SUMMARY

The Gut-Brain Connection

➤ The gut-brain connection is two-directional. Conditions that involve the brain and mood affect digestive function, and, conversely, digestive conditions affect brain and mood function.

➤ As we continue to learn more about how our gut microbes affect our mood, it is clear that probiotics will play an important role in managing or possibly even preventing mood disorders.

Chapter 7

THE SKINNY ON FOOD

Before you convince yourself that you are housing the wrong microbes without a chance of ever regaining your slender shape, know that there is hope. You are not inextricably linked to these bad bugs—you can change your gut balance by eating the right foods. Good gut bacteria thrive on certain foods you eat, while bad bacteria thrive on others. The Standard American Diet (SAD) is high in refined carbohydrates and starches, sugars, and unhealthy fats, and is low in fruits and vegetables, healthy fats, proteins, nuts, and seeds. Thus, SAD is rich in foods that feed the wrong bacteria and low in foods that feed the right bacteria.

Your diet plays a major role in the composition of your gut bacteria, but gut bacteria also affect what you eat. I have always promoted the idea that you cannot address your health without also addressing your dietary habits. Diet is 80 percent of the game. In addition, the contribution of the gut microbes to your nutritional status must be recognized. Your gut bacteria help break down the foods you eat, produce nutrients, and help neutralize toxins in your digestive tract. Each of these factors affects your nutrient status, or how well your body is nourished. If you eat a great diet but your gut is out of balance, you will not fully achieve the health you are capable of enjoying. Conversely, if your gut is in perfect balance, that does not mean you can eat a poor diet and be immune to its negative effects. Indeed, diet and gut balance go hand in hand. Both diet and gut balance need to be addressed to get the kind of changes that will result in weight loss.

That's exactly why I developed the Skinny Gut Diet—so that you can reach your ideal weight by addressing diet and gut balance at the same time.

"The Skinny Gut Diet is the best system of weight loss and getting healthy—inside and out—that I have ever been on." —Dave

Diets high in sugars and refined carbohydrates (which quickly break down into sugars upon digestion) slow the movement of food through the digestive tract and increase the growth of bad bacteria that release toxic compounds. A diet high in saturated fat also increases the production of toxins in the digestive tract. In Chapter 2 you learned that there are toxins known as endotoxins produced by certain bacteria inside the digestive tract. One particular endotoxin is produced by certain gut bacteria, and when combined with a high-fat, high-sugar diet, it triggers silent inflammation that contributes to weight gain and the accumulation of fat.[1] Truly, diet and gut balance go hand in hand.

The effects of diet on gut bacterial balance can occur quickly. That is both good news and bad news, depending on what changes you make to your diet. Switching from a low-fat, high-fiber diet to a high-fat, high-sugar SAD diet has been found to change the gut bacterial composition from a "lean gut type" to an "obese gut type" *within one day*.[2] To change your mix of bacteria for the better, you will want to feed the good bacteria and starve the bad bacteria on a daily basis.

Before we get to the nuts and bolts of the diet, I want you to better understand the foods you eat. Specifically, I want to discuss the macronutrient groups—fats, carbohydrates, and proteins. These three nutrients are what make up the majority of foods we eat. Every day we must eat fats, carbs, and proteins to keep our bodies functioning properly. Unfortunately, some of what we have been told about these nutrients is not entirely accurate. Let's take a closer look.

FAT IS NOT THE ENEMY

You have likely been running from fat most of your life. The idea that fat is the enemy has become so ingrained in our psyches that the very thought of eating a high-fat food makes us feel like we're breaking the rules. I'm here to tell you that what you thought you knew about fat is all wrong. Our bodies need fat to perform a wide array of functions that are necessary for our health. Certain fats are downright healthy; without them we lose our vitality and our health suffers. Consider this: Your brain is about 60 percent fat, and the cells that make up your body are encased in fat. Replenishing those fats through diet is crucial—no question. When you avoid fats, you fail to replenish your body with an essential nutrient.

If you think that fat makes you fat, you might be surprised to learn that sugar and carbohydrates play a greater role in fat accumulation than does fat itself. That's right—a diet high in starchy carbohydrates and sugars directly stimulates the liver to produce fat. That's why many people who eat a diet high in sugar and carbohydrates end up with high triglycerides (fat in the bloodstream).

Not All Fats Are Equal

What I want you to know is that not all fats are created equal. There are two in particular I want you to know about: omega-3 and omega-6 fats. Both omega-3 and omega-6 polyunsaturated fatty acids (or *fats*, for short) are considered essential, meaning they are not produced by the body and must be obtained through the diet. Omega-3 and omega-6 fatty acids make up a significant part of almost all cell membranes—the protective layer surrounding the cell.[3] The SAD diet is plentiful in foods rich in omega-6, but is considered deficient in omega-3–rich foods.

There are a number of reasons for the omega-3/omega-6 imbalance in modern diets. To begin, the introduction of food processing during the Industrial Revolution enabled the widespread production of many foods that previously couldn't be mass produced. Vegetable oil processing was one such introduction, resulting in the mass availability of vegetable oils rich in omega-6. The use of these oils largely replaced the use of butter and, thus, greatly increased the amount of omega-6 fatty acids in the diet, creating a huge imbalance in the omega-3/omega-6 ratio. Add to that the change from a more traditional diet to one that included more processed foods, and there was a general decrease in the total amount of omega-3 consumed, further skewing the omega-3/omega-6 ratio.

> **"This is not a diet. It's a new way of living healthy to feel better, inside and out." —Theresa**

Another result of modern food processing was the mass production of animals for meat consumption. The introduction of grains (high in omega-6 fats) to animal feed, used to fatten the animals, replacing the traditional grass and seeds (high in omega-3 fats) they once ate, has greatly increased the amount of omega-6 fats we consume. Therefore, when we eat these meats, our own omega-3/omega-6 balance becomes further skewed. Additionally, modern agriculture has reduced the omega-3 content of green leafy vegetables, meat, eggs, and even fish.[4] In the hunter-gatherer days, humans ate about the same amount of omega-6s as omega-3s. Today we eat up to twenty-five times more omega-6s than omega-3s.

If you eat foods cooked with the following oils, you are eating a high amount of omega-6 fats:

- Corn oil
- Cottonseed oil
- Vegetable oil
- Safflower oil
- Sunflower oil
- Soybean oil

- Peanut oil
- Shortening

Reducing your omega-6 fat intake by avoiding these oils and cooking with coconut oil and olive oil, along with increasing your intake of beneficial omega-3 fats, will help to reverse the unhealthy omega-3/omega-6 ratio obtained from the Standard American Diet.

On the Skinny Gut Diet you will be eating healthy fats, including:

Cold-pressed olive oil, flaxseed oil, coconut oil
Ghee (clarified butter) or moderate amounts of butter
Foods naturally rich in healthy fats:

Avocados	Pumpkin seeds
Olives	Sunflower seeds
Walnuts	Sardines
Almonds	Salmon
Pecans	Coconut
Flax seeds	Coconut milk
Chia seeds	

When you eat too many omega-6 fats and too few omega-3 fats, your body creates silent inflammation, which you have already learned is an underlying contributor to obesity and chronic disease. To help quell this inflammation, you must be sure to eat the right fats. The Skinny Gut Diet promotes eating healthy fats in the form of fish, nuts, seeds, avocados, and certain oils. You will learn more about what fats to eat in Chapter 9.

What About Saturated Fats?

Saturated fats can be eaten in moderation. A diet very high in saturated fats will feed the bacteria that make you fat, so moderate intake of saturated fats is recommended. But you want to be sure that you replace these fats with *healthy* fats. Fat is an important nutrient that serves many important functions in your body—when you eat the right ones.

Simply put, all saturated fats are not the same. One type of saturated fat that I feel very comfortable with is coconut oil. Coconut oil is high in medium-chain triglycerides (MCTs) while other saturated fats are high in short-chain triglycerides. MCTs are easily digested and rapidly burned for energy, rather than stored like other saturated fats. Coconut oil is also high in lauric acid, a compound that has anti-microbial properties. Due to its high stability, coconut oil is great for cooking.

Olive Oil

You have likely already heard that olive oil is good for you. Rest assured this advice is sound. Olive oil is neither omega-3 nor omega-6, neither saturated fat nor polyunsaturated fat. In a class of its own, olive oil is an omega-9 fat with the highest concentration of mono-unsaturated fat of any edible oil. Olive oil is one of the most heart-healthy oils there is, and therefore is the centerpiece of Mediterranean foods, known for their benefits for the heart. Extra-virgin olive oil is particularly healthy, best reserved for uncooked foods such as salads and dips.

CARBS—THE MYTH OF HEALTHY WHOLE GRAINS

You may be surprised to learn that grains are not the health food they are made out to be. Grains are now recognized as inflammatory foods, for a number of reasons. A diet high in grains—whole or refined—promotes gut imbalance, increases leaky gut, and raises blood sugar and insulin levels, among other negative health effects, all of which increase inflammation. In fact—and I learned this from my friend, the amazing Dr. William Davis of *Wheat Belly* fame—two slices of whole wheat bread raise blood sugar more than do two tablespoons of pure sugar. So much for healthy whole grains. I'm here to tell you that you don't need these foods. It's time to end this energy-sucking, health-depleting relationship—your love affair with grains—before it becomes disastrous.

Before you go into shock at this news, know that there are substitutions you can make that allow you to enjoy some of the grain-containing foods you are accustomed to. Non-grain flours and low-carb pasta are just two of many foods that you can still enjoy on the Skinny Gut Diet. The carbohydrates you will eat on the Skinny Gut Diet come from nonstarchy vegetables, low-sugar fruits, nuts, seeds, and dairy. Not only are these foods packed with nutrients, they are also high in fiber to fuel your good bacteria. You will learn more about these foods in Chapter 9. But first, an important word on gluten—one carb I feel strongly about.

Gluten Gut

By removing grains from your diet, you will effectively be removing gluten, a protein found in wheat, barley, rye, and in some oats, due to cross-contamination. Removing grains is a good thing, since wheat and gluten are known to trigger a wide range of symptoms and health conditions, and are closely tied to weight gain.

Fortunately, it is easier than ever to find gluten-free alternatives. Your best bet will be to seek out foods that are labeled "gluten free," but you can also read ingredient labels to determine whether a food is made with gluten. (If it's not labeled "gluten free" it may still contain traces of gluten from cross-contamination during manufacturing. I'll let you decide how strict you want to be.) The following is a list of ingredients that indicate the food contains wheat or gluten:

- Barley
- Breading and bread stuffing
- Brewer's yeast
- Bulgur wheat

- Durum wheat
- Farro/faro
- Graham flour (whole wheat flour)
- Hydrolyzed wheat protein
- Kamut
- Malt, malt extract, malt syrup, and malt flavoring
- Malt vinegar
- Malted milk
- Matzoh, matzoh meal
- Modified wheat starch
- Oatmeal, oat bran, oat flour, and whole oats (unless labeled "gluten free")
- Rye bread and rye flour
- Seitan
- Semolina
- Spelt
- Triticale
- Wheat bran
- Wheat flour
- Wheat germ
- Wheat starch

As much as possible, try to avoid foods that contain these ingredients. Sauces and seasonings—as well as most processed, packaged foods—are the most common sources of hidden gluten. Read the label to be sure.

> Always remember that "gluten-free" does not mean
> sugar-free. Be sure to read your labels.
> Often, gluten-free foods contain more sugar and starchy
> carbohydrates than their wheat counterparts.

A primary goal of the Skinny Gut Diet is to balance your gut. Research (and experience) shows that starchy carbohydrates (potatoes, grains, pastas, breads, etc.) and sugars increase inflammation and lead to gut imbalance and obesity. Before you fret about having to give up your favorite foods, please know that the Skinny Gut Diet is full of delicious foods you can eat that will take away your cravings—and your extra weight. In Chapter 9 you will learn about what foods you will be eating, and in Chapter 13 you will find a variety of delicious, easy-to-prepare recipes to keep you inspired, well fed, and skinny.

A Word on Fiber

Fiber is your friend, for three main reasons:

1. It doesn't break down into absorbable sugar.
2. It slows the absorption of sugar from other foods.
3. It acts as food for your good gut bacteria.

> **"I have found my super fruit fiber supplement to be a satisfying product when used to curb my sweet cravings. I sprinkle it in my shakes, in my plain yogurt with berries, and even in my veggie juice." —Cynthia**

The Skinny Gut Diet includes plenty of high-fiber vegetables and fruits, but you would be amazed at how much you have to eat in order to reach the recommended daily intake of 35 grams. Even if you absolutely love your veggies, you would be hard pressed to reach this goal every day without serious effort (and chewing). Fortunately, there is an easy way to reach your daily fiber goal without eating salad for breakfast, lunch, and dinner. Fiber supplements are an excellent way to do just that—supplement your diet. A high-quality fiber supplement is a recommended Skinny Gut supplement, discussed in Chapter 11.

SKINNY GUT DIET SUCCESS STORY: ALEXANDRA A.

Alexandra is an extraordinary 25-year-old woman. She is raising her 15-year-old brother while holding down a full-time job as an administrative assistant, all while recently completing a year of physical and occupational therapy training at her local hospital on weekends. She also enjoys a very stable and loving relationship with her boyfriend of six years. At her young age, she is truly a person to admire.

Alexandra has a natural curiosity about nutrition and health, and has been educating herself for years. Prior to the Skinny Gut Diet program, she found herself frustrated by her inability to lose weight and keep it off, despite her best efforts to work out. She told me that she often felt exhausted and mentally foggy. Life seemed difficult at times.

When she began the Skinny Gut Diet program, Alexandra tended toward constipation, although she hadn't considered her poor bowel habits to be a health concern, as is the case with so many people. (One great thing about the Skinny Gut Diet is that you will learn how important it is to move your bowels regularly; your health will be so much better when you do.) On the diet, though, Alexandra was able to overcome her chronic constipation. In addition, developing consistent eating habits has been a key to her success. Consuming protein every few hours has quieted her ravenous cravings.

Avoiding wheat and gluten has also been very helpful for Alexandra. It is likely that she has a gluten sensitivity, although she hasn't been officially tested. The clue was her unforgettable digestive experience when she splurged on chocolate chip cookies. It took her days to return to normal. She tells me that she is not likely to splurge again.

It has always amazed me how rapidly my own body tells me what is good and not good for me once I clean up my habits and pay attention. So many people go through their lives never experiencing how a healthy body feels because food sensitivities keep them constantly at odds with their bodies, unbeknownst to them. They don't feel good, but they don't recognize that they feel bad. The contrast is not stark. These people fall somewhere between feeling mediocre and just getting by, all the while accepting their suffering as normal. Poor health is not normal! You will begin to understand this once you have immersed yourself in Skinny Gut living.

"My energy level since the beginning of the Skinny Gut Diet has been remarkable. I no longer feel exhausted or foggy. I feel new, and I enjoy shrinking without starving myself." —Alexandra

Alexandra looks and feels fabulous after letting go of 22 pounds. Her goal is to double that, and she is well on her way. The Skinny Gut Diet is helping Alexandra better understand her body and has ignited a passion in her for sharing the information with others. Already her boyfriend and brother have shifted their eating patterns, and her boyfriend has lost some weight, too. A career in nutrition may be beckoning. I am certainly filled with encouragement. I know how rewarding it is to see lives change simply through understanding good gut health.

Alexandra	Weight	Waistline Inches	Body Fat %
Before	187	36½"	35.8%
After	165	33½"	34.9%
Lost	22 lbs.	3"	0.9%

PROTEIN AND APPETITE CONTROL

Protein is your ally when fighting cravings or hunger pangs, especially when you begin to change your intake of carbohydrates. Protein is an important component of a successful weight-loss diet, and helps to balance blood sugar. It's helpful to have a high-protein snack close by if you're hit with cravings for sugary or starchy foods. You would be amazed at how eating protein every two to three hours will subdue your cravings.

> **"Unlike other diets, I feel like I am constantly eating and yet I am still losing weight. I have learned a great deal about protein, and how it helps to control sugar cravings. This program has been a great help in my daily life." —Alexandra**

Breakfast is one meal that can quickly turn your plate into a carb fest if you fall into the old habits. Pancakes, muffins, cereals, French toast, crepes, doughnuts—sometimes breakfast resembles dessert more than it does a well-balanced meal. It's no wonder your cravings kick in mid-morning. On the Skinny Gut Diet, you will start your day off with plenty of protein. Studies have found that a high-protein breakfast makes you feel full longer.[5] Eating protein at breakfast is essential for avoiding carb cravings later.

Meal-Replacement Shakes on the Go

If your calendar is full—and whose isn't?—you will be glad to hear that there is an effortless way to keep your protein intake up while not being held hostage in your kitchen. Meal-replacement shakes are naturally high in protein and nutrients, and they can double as a meal when you need it or as a snack to keep you going strong. Look for a high-quality meal replacement that contains 20 grams of protein and 10 grams of fiber per serving, along with an array of vitamins and minerals to keep your energy high and your cravings low. See Chapter 10 for more about meal-replacement shakes as snacks or an occasional meal.

Stay Hydrated

Throughout the day, preferably between meals, drink half your weight in ounces of purified water. (The amount is determined by dividing your body weight—using pounds rather than kilograms—by 2.) For example, a 160-pound person would need to drink 80 ounces (2½ quarts) of water daily. Good hydration is important to the function of every cell in your body. Water helps rid your body of toxins via improved bowel movements and kidney function. Half of your body is water, so you want to replenish this vital resource so that you will function at your best.

If you do not like drinking plain water, you can drink herbal tea, fruit- or vegetable-infused waters, sparkling water, vegetable juice (see drink recipes in Chapter 10), or beverages sweetened with natural, non-calorie sweeteners such as stevia or erythritol. Caffeinated drinks do not count as part of your daily water intake, however, because they have dehydrating properties. That does not mean you can't have your coffee or tea. You will not have to give up your morning cup of joe on the Skinny Gut Diet—just the sugar you add to it.

SKINNY GUT DIET SUCCESS STORY: DANIELLE A.

Danielle is a lovely 30-year-old woman with a full-time career as a business analyst and who has a 7-year-old son and a loving husband (who previously enjoyed whatever food she put in front of him or picked up at a drive-through). Both Danielle and her spouse had battled their weight for years. As the years of their marriage accumulated, so did the pounds. It didn't seem to matter that Danielle worked out vigorously four or five times weekly. She had tried myriad diet plans, but nothing seemed to work. More and more, she felt exhausted and unenthused.

Danielle is one of the most organized, detail-oriented women I've had the pleasure to meet. When she began the Skinny Gut Diet, she told me that she was sometimes angry with herself for not being able to handle her weight more effectively. This woman had put a lot of effort into dieting in the past, to no avail. Danielle also told me that she had frequent stomach pains, but she had no idea why. In addition, she had been told that her cholesterol was a bit high—at 30 years old!

What fun it has been to watch 30 pounds drop off Danielle as she reached her goal through the Skinny Gut lifestyle. She was astounded to experience her cravings vanish while her energy increased. She no longer felt exhausted. Importantly, her stomach pains were gone. All of these benefits make the Skinny Gut Diet more than simply a diet. It's an eating plan for life. Feeling this good will give you the motivation to change for the better—and it's so easy.

Notably, on the Skinny Gut Diet, Danielle's Fat bacteria decreased and her Be Skinny bacteria increased.

ADIPOSITY INDEX
DANIELLE

BEFORE:

Expected Value

Firmicutes % **51**		< = 80%
Bacteroidetes % **49**		> = 20%

AFTER:

Expected Value

Firmicutes % **42**		< = 80%
Bacteroidetes % **58**		> = 20%

"Before the Skinny Gut Diet I had tried so many diets. I worked out regularly, but didn't see any results. This continued for years. I wondered if it was just me—maybe I wasn't meant to be the proper size for my height. Within the first month of starting the diet, I was seeing so many improvements—not only with my body, but with my mind. I look at food differently now." —Danielle

Remember Danielle's husband? Well, he also lost 25 pounds as a result of adopting some of Danielle's eating habits. And he reports that he is now able to have pain-free bowel movements, something he had suffered for years. He says that he feels 100 times better, and he isn't even following all aspects of the diet. Once Danielle understood the why and the how, she simply led by example. She didn't allow anyone to influence her behaviors, and as a result, the gifts in her life keep multiplying.

Danielle	Weight	Waistline Inches	Body Fat %
Before	184	35"	36.8%
After	154	30½"	32.8%
Lost	30 lbs	4½"	4.0%

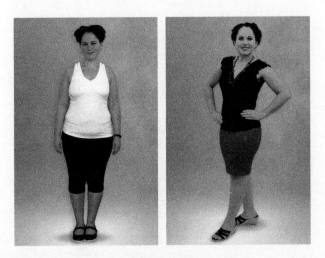

Before and After

CHAPTER 7 SUMMARY

Eating for a Skinny Gut

➤ Our bodies need fat to perform a wide array of functions that are necessary for our health. Certain fats are downright healthy; without them we lose our vitality, and our health suffers.

➤ Grains are not the health food they are made out to be. The carbohydrates you will eat on the Skinny Gut Diet do not come from grains, but instead come from nonstarchy vegetables, low-sugar fruits, nuts, seeds, and dairy.

➤ Protein is your ally when fighting cravings or hunger pangs, especially when you begin to change your intake of carbohydrates.

➤ Meal replacement shakes are naturally high in protein, fiber, and nutrients and can double as a meal when you need it to or as a snack to keep you going strong.

➤ Good hydration is important to the function of every cell in your body. You will want to drink half of your body weight in ounces of water daily.

Chapter 8

TEASPOON TRACKER

As I mentioned in Chapter 2, the Skinny Gut Diet is made up of three simple rules that will help you balance your gut and lose weight for good. I will get to those rules in the next chapter, but first I want to introduce you to a tool that will bring everything together for you. My Teaspoon Tracker will help you learn how to eat the right foods in a way that changes your whole perspective on eating, especially when it comes to hidden sugar. By applying my Teaspoon Tracker to the three simple rules of the Skinny Gut Diet, you will be prepared to eat delicious foods that will help you reclaim your skinny gut.

DEFINITION

Teaspoons of sugar: When I refer to the teaspoons of sugar contained in the foods you eat, I am not only talking about the added and natural sugars found in foods but also the starches that are found in carbohydrates, which are converted into sugar in your digestive tract and are absorbed as sugar by the body. I consider these starches to be "hidden sugars" because you won't find them listed as sugar on food labels.

Carbohydrates break down into sugars in your digestive tract so that the body can absorb those sugars to use as fuel. The problem is that the body does not need nearly as much sugar as it gets from the Standard American Diet. In fact, the body needs only the equivalent of *1 teaspoon of sugar in the bloodstream at any time*. Yet the average American consumes at least 37 teaspoons of sugar daily—that's far too much. And if that average American eats a fast-food diet, he could easily be ingesting 86 teaspoons of sugar daily. When you're eating this much sugar, the harmful bacteria in your gut flourish, and you hold onto excess weight. If you overload your sugar intake (including the hidden sugars from starchy carbohydrates), your body works overtime to deal with it. Maintaining a healthy daily intake of sugar—from all foods—is a crucial part of balancing both your gut and your metabolism.

There are basically three types of carbohydrates—starch, sugar, and fiber. Starch breaks down into sugar in the digestive tract, sugar remains as is and is readily absorbed by the body, and fiber resists digestion, passing through the digestive tract largely intact. As you have learned, the friendly bacteria in your gut dine on fiber, especially soluble fiber, which you will find plentiful in the Skinny Gut Diet.

The Teaspoon Tracker

Here's a unique calculation that helps you track the teaspoons of sugar (including hidden sugar) in the foods you eat. And you'll need only look at the total carbohydrates and dietary fiber in that food:

$$\left(\begin{array}{c}\text{TOTAL}\\\text{CARBOHYDRATES}\end{array} - \text{DIETARY FIBER}\right) \div 5 = \begin{array}{c}\text{TEASPOONS}\\\text{OF SUGAR}\end{array}$$

Total carbohydrates minus dietary fiber, divided by 5 gives you the total teaspoons of sugar contained in your food. This simple calculation will help you determine how much sugar is *really* in the foods you eat. By subtracting the fiber from the carbohydrates, you reveal the total grams of sugar plus starchy carbohydrates. From there, you simply divide by 5 to convert to teaspoons of sugar (because there are about 5 grams in 1 teaspoon of sugar). It's that easy. I like this calculation because it is easier to visualize teaspoons than grams. And sometimes it's scary how many teaspoons of sugar are in our foods!

NOTE

Be careful not to confuse the teaspoons of sugar from this calculation with the grams of sugar found on Nutrition Facts panels on food packaging. The grams measure accounts for the added sugar and the sugars found naturally in foods, but not the sugars that come from the breakdown of starches. You can essentially ignore the sugar reading on the Nutrition Facts panel. Rely on the Teaspoon Tracker instead.

Let's try this out, using some Nutrition Facts panels, shall we? You know the grid—the list of nutrient amounts on packaged foods. The label below shows the nutrients in a medium-sized banana.

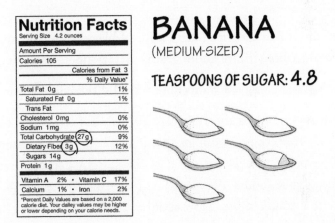

Nutrition Facts

Serving Size 4.2 ounces

Amount Per Serving

Calories 105

	Calories from Fat 3
	% Daily Value*
Total Fat 0g	1%
Saturated Fat 0g	1%
Trans Fat	
Cholesterol 0mg	0%
Sodium 1mg	0%
Total Carbohydrate 27g	9%
Dietary Fiber 3g	12%
Sugars 14g	
Protein 1g	
Vitamin A 2% • Vitamin C 17%	
Calcium 1% • Iron 2%	

*Percent Daily Values are based on a 2,000 calorie diet. Your dailey values may be higher or lower depending on your calorie needs.

BANANA
(MEDIUM-SIZED)

TEASPOONS OF SUGAR: 4.8

You can see that a banana contains 27 grams of carbohydrates and 3 grams of fiber. Let's plug it into the formula:

27 grams carbs – 3 grams fiber ÷ 5 = 4.8 teaspoons sugar

Bananas are a high-sugar fruit, as you can see. You would think from looking at the Nutrition Facts panel that the banana contains less than 3 teaspoons of sugar (14 grams of sugar divided by 5 = 2.8), but you wouldn't be taking into account the hidden sugars found in the starch. My formula helps you find those hidden sugars so you know the truth about what you are eating.

Let's try another fruit. How about blackberries?

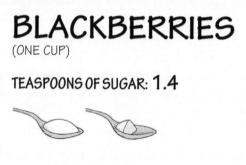

Nutrition Facts
Serving Size 5.1 ounces

Amount Per Serving

Calories 62

Calories from Fat 6

% Daily Value*

Total Fat 0g	1%
Saturated Fat 0g	0%
Trans Fat	
Cholesterol 0mg	0%
Sodium 1mg	0%
Total Carbohydrate 15g	5%
Dietary Fiber 8g	31%
Sugars 7g	
Protein 2g	

Vitamin A	6%	Vitamin C	50%
Calcium	4%	Iron	5%

*Percent Daily Values are based on a 2,000 calorie diet. Your dailey values may be higher or lower depending on your calorie needs.

BLACKBERRIES
(ONE CUP)

TEASPOONS OF SUGAR: 1.4

One cup of blackberries (that's a lot of blackberries!) contains 15 grams total carbohydrates and 8 grams dietary fiber. Let's plug it in:

15 grams carbs – 8 grams fiber ÷ 5 = 1.4 teaspoons sugar

One full cup of blackberries contains only 1.4 teaspoons of sugar. You can see from these examples that it also helps to have more fiber. Fiber essentially cancels out some of the starchy carbohydrates and sugars from your foods.

Let's do a couple more. How about brown rice?

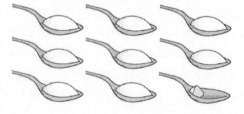

Nutrition Facts
Serving Size 7 ounces

Amount Per Serving

Calories 218

Calories from Fat 14

% Daily Value*

Total Fat 2g	2%
Saturated Fat 0g	2%
Trans Fat	
Cholesterol 0mg	0%
Sodium 2mg	0%
Total Carbohydrate 46g	15%
Dietary Fiber 4g	14%
Sugars	
Protein 5g	

Vitamin A	0%	Vitamin C	0%
Calcium	2%	Iron	6%

*Percent Daily Values are based on a 2,000 calorie diet. Your dailey values may be higher or lower depending on your calorie needs.

BROWN RICE
(ONE CUP, COOKED)

TEASPOONS OF SUGAR: 8.2

One cup of cooked brown rice contains 46 grams of total carbohydrates and 4 grams dietary fiber. Let's plug it in:

45 grams carbs – 4 grams fiber ÷ 5 = 8.2 teaspoons sugar

Wow! Now that's an eye-opener. Brown rice is considered a healthy whole grain, but in the body it breaks down into more than 8 teaspoons of sugar, owing to its high starch content. Brown rice is not the only culprit here, either. Other grains—such as the highly lauded quinoa—are also high in sugar. That's why grains are not included in the GET LEAN PHASE of the Skinny Gut Diet. In the STAY LEAN PHASE, you will add back some of these foods in moderation.

Now let's look at cooked spinach.

SPINACH
(COOKED)

Nutrition Facts

Serving Size 6.4 ounces

Amount Per Serving

Calories 41

	Calories from Fat 4
	% Daily Value*
Total Fat 0g	1%
Saturated Fat 0g	0%
Trans Fat	
Cholesterol 0mg	0%
Sodium 126mg	5%
Total Carbohydrate 7g	2%
Dietary Fiber 4g	17%
Sugars 1g	
Protein 5g	

Vitamin A 377%	•	Vitamin C 29%
Calcium 24%	•	Iron 36%

*Percent Daily Values are based on a 2,000 calorie diet. Your dailey values may be higher or lower depending on your calorie needs.

TEASPOONS OF SUGAR: 0.6

One cup of cooked spinach contains 7 grams carbohydrates and 4 grams dietary fiber. Let's plug it in:

7 grams carbs – 4 grams fiber ÷ 5 = 0.6 teaspoons sugar

Like most nonstarchy vegetables, green leafy vegetables such as spinach are the stars of the Skinny Gut Diet. Not only are they packed with nutrients—green leafy vegetables are among the most nutrient-dense foods around—but they are also high in fiber and low in sugar.

Now it's your turn to practice so that you get familiar with this calculation and can apply it when you are shopping. The following Nutrition Facts panel is for one doughnut. Fill in the blanks to arrive at your total teaspoons of sugar.

Nutrition Facts
Serving Size One 4.5 inch Doughnut

Amount Per Serving

Calories 299   Calories from Fat 129

% Daily Value*

Total Fat 14g	22%
Saturated Fat 4g	20%
Trans Fat	
Cholesterol 23mg	6%
Sodium 290mg	12%
Total Carbohydrate 38g	13%
Dietary Fiber 2g	6%
Sugars 15g	
Protein 5g	

Vitamin A 0% • Vitamin C 1%
Calcium 3% • Iron 16%

*Percent Daily Values are based on a 2,000 calorie diet. Your dailey values may be higher or lower depending on your calorie needs.

DOUGHNUT
(ONE)

TEASPOONS OF SUGAR: _____

___ grams carbs – ___ grams fiber ÷ 5 = ___ teaspoons sugar

Wow. You might want to pass on your next doughnut. Now let's try another one. The following is a Nutrition Facts panel for plain Greek yogurt.

Nutrition Facts
Serving Size 6oz (170g)

Amount Per Serving

Calories 100   Calories from Fat 0

% Daily Value*

Total Fat 0g	0%
Saturated Fat 0g	0%
Trans Fat 0g	
Cholesterol 0mg	0%
Sodium 80mg	3%
Total Carbohydrate 7g	2%
Dietary Fiber 0g	6%
Sugars 7g	
Protein 18g	36%

Vitamin A 0% • Vitamin C 0%
Calcium 20% • Iron 0%

*Percent Daily Values are based on a 2,000 calorie diet. Your dailey values may be higher or lower depending on your calorie needs.

GREEK YOGURT
(PLAIN)

TEASPOONS OF SUGAR: _____

___ grams carbs – ___ grams fiber ÷ 5 = ___ teaspoons sugar

As you can see, plain Greek yogurt is a much better option than a doughnut for breakfast. Not only do you get much less total sugar and carbohydrate, but you also get an excellent amount of protein. Add some low-sugar fruit for flavor. A little bit goes a long way.

Carbohydrates are a very misunderstood food group. Yes, our bodies need carbohydrates. Carbohydrates break down into glucose (sugar), which is used for energy by every cell in your body. However, we get far more carbohydrates than our body needs to maintain its energy levels. First, consider the added sugars—they are so abundant in the diet and are literally sickening the nation. The Skinny Gut Diet eliminates added sugars as much as possible. They are simply not necessary in the diet and only contribute to poor health.

But even if you eliminate all added sugars from your diet, you will still be consuming large amounts of hidden sugars in grains, potatoes, many fruits, and even beans. Starchy carbohydrates break down into sugar, all the same. In case you haven't noticed, those foods—especially grains, which are very high in hidden sugars—can trigger cravings every bit as strong as sugar triggers. Now you know why. The Teaspoon Tracker is critical when you are trying to lose weight. Understanding this concept and being able to apply it when you eat are vital.

CHAPTER 8 SUMMARY

By applying my Teaspoon Tracker to the three simple rules of the Skinny Gut Diet, you will be prepared to eat delicious foods that will help you reclaim your skinny gut.

➤ There are basically three types of carbohydrates—starch, sugar, and fiber. Starch breaks down into sugar in the digestive tract, sugar remains as is and is readily absorbed by the body, and fiber resists digestion, passing through the digestive tract largely intact.

➤ My unique Teaspoon Tracker formula will help you track the teaspoons of sugar (including hidden sugar) in the foods you eat. You need only look at the total carbohydrates and dietary fiber in your food:

$$\left(\begin{array}{c} \text{TOTAL} \\ \text{CARBOHYDRATES} \end{array} - \text{DIETARY FIBER} \right) \div 5 = \begin{array}{c} \text{TEASPOONS} \\ \text{OF SUGAR} \end{array}$$

➤ Total carbohydrates minus dietary fiber, divided by 5 gives you the total teaspoons of sugar contained in your food. This simple tool will help you determine how much sugar is *really* in the foods you eat.

Be careful not to confuse the teaspoons of sugar calculated from the Teaspoon Tracker with the grams of sugar found on Nutrition Facts panels on food packaging, which account for the added sugar and the sugars found naturally in foods, but not the sugars that come from the breakdown of starches.

Chapter 9

THE GET LEAN PHASE

You have already taken a big step in a healthy direction. You are embarking on a journey that is much more than a diet. It's a new way of eating. And it's simple once you make it a habit. The Skinny Gut Diet is not about what you can't eat; it's about what you *can* eat. Many people are struggling with weight gain, not because they can't stick to a healthy diet and lifestyle, not because they are lazy, and not because they have the wrong genes. They struggle with dieting because they are not taking into account the gut factor. If the gut is out of balance, lasting weight loss cannot be achieved. The Skinny Gut Diet addresses the gut factor by balancing your gut so that you can achieve—and maintain—your healthy weight.

The Skinny Gut Diet includes foods that feed the beneficial bacteria in your gut and that support your digestive health. The focus is on moving away from eating foods that feed harmful bacteria and welcoming a diet rich in foods that balance your gut. As a result, you will lose the weight you have been carrying around for years, literally and figuratively.

The Skinny Gut Diet is divided into two phases:
1. GET LEAN PHASE
2. STAY LEAN PHASE

You will remain in the GET LEAN PHASE until you have reached your desired weight, at which point you will switch to the STAY LEAN PHASE, designed to help you fine-tune your eating

habits and personalize your diet for your body. I developed the STAY
LEAN PHASE to be flexible because everyone is unique. Both
phases are made up of three simple rules:

Rule 1: Eat more fat (*healthy* fat) to reduce silent inflammation.
Rule 2: Eat living foods every day to balance your gut.
Rule 3: Eat protein at every meal and snack to eliminate cravings.

The Skinny Gut Diet is not complicated. You won't have to ven-
ture through three or more phases, wondering what you'll be doing
next or if you're in the right phase. The rules are straightforward and
easy to follow. That's because I want you to get comfortable with
eating this way so that it sticks. Once you get used to eating healthy
fats, proteins, and plenty of living foods, you will look and feel great.

And I want you to look and feel great for life. That's why I designed the diet so that you will be able to incorporate these concepts
without going back to the book every day for help. Sure, the first
month or so you will need to refer back to these pages as you incorporate my three simple rules, but you will soon get a feel for how to eat
on your own. That's the beauty of this diet. You will be creating new
habits to replace your old habits—for life.

GET LEAN PHASE: EAT 8 TO 10 TEASPOONS OF SUGAR DAILY.

During the GET LEAN PHASE, you will set your target to consume between 8 and 10 teaspoons of sugar from *all* the foods you eat
(including hidden sugar) daily. This will be your overarching goal
while you follow the three simple rules, and it is the crux of the diet.
Using my unique Teaspoon Tracker calculation will help you stay on
track.

$$\left(\frac{\text{TOTAL}}{\text{CARBOHYDRATES}} - \text{DIETARY FIBER}\right) \div 5 = \text{TEASPOONS OF SUGAR}$$

RULE I
EAT MORE FAT (*HEALTHY* FAT) TO REDUCE SILENT INFLAMMATION

You have already learned from Chapter 7 that fat is not the enemy. Healthy fats—especially those high in omega-3 fats—will help to quell the silent inflammation that comes with being overweight. On the Skinny Gut Diet you will not have to track your fat intake. Instead, you will simply make sure that you are eating the right fats while avoiding the wrong ones.

Fats to Enjoy

- Cold-pressed olive oil, flaxseed oil, coconut oil
- Ghee (clarified butter) or moderate amounts of butter
- Foods naturally rich in healthy fats:

Avocados	Pumpkin seeds
Olives	Sunflower seeds
Walnuts	Sardines
Almonds	Salmon
Pecans	Coconut
Flax seeds	Coconut milk
Chia seeds	

Fats to Avoid

Trans fats	Sunflower oil
Corn oil	Soybean oil
Cottonseed oil	Peanut oil
Vegetable oil	Shortening
Safflower oil	

How Much Fat?

On the Skinny Gut Diet you do not need to keep track of your fat intake. Fat is not the evil health destroyer it was once promoted to be. Much of the fat you will be getting will be beneficial fat. How much saturated fat, you might ask? Most saturated fat will come from meat and dairy products. You can have lean, preferably grass-fed red meat up to three times per week. (Keep in mind that a serving of meat is 4 to 6 ounces, about the size of the palm of your hand.) And yes, you can have full-fat dairy—in moderation. As for coconut oil, because the saturated fat in coconut oil is a medium-chain triglyceride and does not get stored as fat as readily as other saturated fats, you do not have to limit your use of coconut oil. In fact, coconut oil is a perfect cooking oil.

RULE 2

EAT LIVING FOODS EVERY DAY TO BALANCE YOUR GUT

In the Skinny Gut Diet, *living foods* include those foods that increase your good gut bacteria. The living foods that you will eat daily include the following:

- Fermented foods
- Nonstarchy vegetables
- Low-sugar fruits

Living foods either contain beneficial bacteria or they act as food for the beneficial bacteria already in the gut. When you eat living foods on a regular basis, you will replenish the good bacteria in your gut, and you will increase your fiber intake, which helps control your appetite. Now let's look at each of these categories.

Fermented Foods—Delicious and Nutritious

Every day, you will eat a minimum of one serving of fermented foods. Fermented foods are rich in good bacteria that help keep your gut in balance and your waistline whittled. When foods are fermented, beneficial bacteria—those either naturally present in the food or added—begin to break down the foods in a process that creates distinct and various flavors depending on the food, the bacteria involved, and the length of time the food is fermented. As a result, fermented foods are easier to digest. You can think of fermented foods as being predigested and full of billions of good bacteria. See Chapter 13 for a homemade sauerkraut (fermented vegetable) recipe (page 217) so that you can prepare your own fermented foods, and see Resources, page 256, for recommended books and packaged fermented foods available for purchase.

Fermented foods include the following:

Live cultured pickles
Sauerkraut
Cultured vegetables
Kimchi
Cheese made from raw milk
Unpasteurized miso
Tempeh
Kombucha
Yogurt containing live cultures
Kefir (dairy and nondairy)

Enjoy Your Prebiotics—Food for Probiotics

In addition to fermented foods, you will eat plenty of foods rich in soluble fibers called prebiotics, which feed the good bacteria in your gut. Aim to include these high-prebiotic foods in your diet as often as possible.

Common foods rich in prebiotics include the following:

Jerusalem artichokes (sunchokes)	Leeks
	Onions
Dandelion greens	Asparagus
Garlic	

You will also eat plenty of other nonstarchy vegetables and low-sugar fruits, which naturally contain soluble fiber and will help to feed the beneficial bacteria in your gut, not to mention provide loads of nutrients that will keep you at your healthiest. How much in the way of fruits and veggies? Eat as many nonstarchy vegetables and low-sugar fruits as possible. Set your goal to eat between five and nine servings each day. At least one of these servings will be fermented vegetables. Soluble prebiotic fiber is a critical part of increasing the beneficial bacteria in your gut, which is why I also recommend that you take a soluble fiber supplement (see Chapter 11).

How to Choose Fruits and Vegetables

Get familiar with the wide variety of nonstarchy vegetables and low-sugar fruits that you will be able to enjoy. The following lists will help guide your choices when it comes to filling your plate with the right foods.

QUICK AND EASY FRUIT CHOICES

Choose either two from column A or one from column B each day. This will add approximately 2.5 teaspoons of sugar to your daily total.

A: FRUITS TO ENJOY — tsp sugar

0 to 1 teaspoon sugar

	tsp sugar
Lychee, 1	0.4
Apricot, 1	0.6
Blackberries, ½ cup	0.7
Cranberries, raw, ½ cup	0.7
Raspberries, ½ cup	0.7
Carambola (star fruit), 1	1.0
Guava, 1	1.0
Lime, 1	1.0
Strawberries, ½ cup	1.0

1 to 1.5 teaspoons sugar

	tsp sugar
Cherries, sour, ½ cup	1.1
Papaya, ½ cup	1.1
Lemon, 1	1.2
Plum, 1 medium	1.4

B: FRUITS TO ENJOY — tsp sugar

1.5 to 2 teaspoons sugar

	tsp sugar
Apple, Granny Smith, ½ large	1.6
Cantaloupe, 1 wedge	1.6
Blueberries, ½ cup	1.7
Grapefruit, white, ½ large	1.8
Apple, 1½ large	1.9
Cherries, sweet, ½ cup	1.9
Kiwifruit, 1 large	2.0
Pineapple, ½ cup	2.0

2 to 2.5 teaspoons sugar

	tsp sugar
Grapefruit, pink, ½ large	2.2

FRUITS TO AVOID — tsp sugar

2.5 to 3 teaspoons sugar

	tsp sugar
Pomegranate, ½ cup	2.6
Honeydew melon, 1 wedge	2.8
Tangerine, 1 large	2.8

3.5 to 4 teaspoons sugar

	tsp sugar
Orange, 1 large	3.6

FRUITS TO AVOID — tsp sugar

4 to 5 teaspoons sugar

	tsp sugar
Watermelon, 2 cups diced	4.0
Banana, 1 medium	4.8
Mango, ½ cup	5.0

5+ teaspoons sugar

	tsp sugar
Pear, 1 large	5.8
Plantain, 1	10.6

QUICK AND EASY VEGETABLE CHOICES

Choose at least five per day. This will add approximately 2.5 teaspoons of sugar to your daily total.*

A: VEGETABLES TO ENJOY   tsp sugar

0 to 0.5 teaspoons sugar

Chives, 1 tablespoon	0
Endive, ½ cup	0
Watercress, 1 cup	0
Cabbage, ½ cup shredded	0.1
Celery, 1 stalk	0.1
Cucumber, ½ cup	0.2
Nopales, ½ cup	0.1
Spinach, 1 cups raw	0.1
Asparagus, ½ cup	0.2
Bamboo sprouts	0.2
Cauliflower, ½ cup	0.2
Eggplant, ½ cup`	0.2
Lettuce, 1 cup	0.2
Radicchio, ½ cup	0.2
Radish, ½ cup	0.2
Tomatillo, 1	0.2
Artichoke hearts, ½ cup	0.3
Arugula, 2 cups	0.3
Chard, ½ cup cooked	0.3
Fennel, ½ cup	0.3
Hearts of palm, ½ cup canned	0.3
Kohlrabi, ½ cup	0.3
Squash, summer yellow, ½ cup	0.3
Squash, zucchini, ½ cup	0.3

A: VEGETABLES TO ENJOY   tsp sugar

0 to 0.5 teaspoons sugar (cont.)

Bean sprouts, ½ cup	0.4
Beans, green, ½ cup	0.4
Broccoli, ½ cup	0.4
Collards, ½ cup cooked	0.4
Kale, ½ cup cooked	0.4
Mushrooms, ½ cup	0.4
Okra, ½ cup	0.4
Snow peas/snap peas, ½ cup	0.4
Shallot, 1 tablespoon	0.4
Brussels sprouts, ½ cup	0.5
Jicama, ½ cup	0.5

0.5 to 1 teaspoon of sugar

Hot peppers	0.2 to 0.6
Leek, ¼ cup	0.6
Onions, ¼ cup	0.6
Turnip, ½ cup	0.6
Pumpkin, ½ cup	0.7
Rutabaga, ½ cup	0.7
Squash, spaghetti, ½ cup	0.7
Avocado, 1	0.8
Carrots, ½ cup	0.8
Beets, ½ cup	0.9
Bell pepper, green, 1 large	1.0
Tomato, red, 1 large	1.0

B: VEGETABLES TO ENJOY   tsp sugar

1 to 1.5 teaspoons sugar

Squash, acorn, ½ cup	1.3
Squash, butternut, ½ cup	1.3
Green peas, ½ cup	1.4
Tomato, green, 1 large	1.4

B: VEGETABLES TO ENJOY   tsp sugar

1.5 to 2 teaspoons sugar

Edamame, ½ cup	1.7
Red/yellow pepper, 1 large	2.0

2 to 2.5 teaspoons sugar

Sweet potato, ½ cup	2.3

B: VEGETABLES TO AVOID	tsp sugar	VEGETABLES TO AVOID	tsp sugar
3.5 to 5 teaspoons of sugar		**5+ teaspoons of sugar**	
Yam, ½ cup	3.6	Cassava (yucca), ½ cup	7.4
Corn, 1 large ear	4.6	Parsnips, ½ cup	8.5
		Potato, 1 large	10.0

*All measures are for raw vegetables unless otherwise specified.

If you like to do the math yourself, you can see that even if you reach nine servings of fruits and vegetables per day, that doesn't mean you will be consuming a lot of sugar.

If you are like me, you like visuals: they make the point clearer. That's why I give you the following chart to help you to visualize what ½ cup of broccoli or 2 cups of salad looks like.

PORTION	VISUAL
¼ cup	an egg/Ping-Pong ball
½ cup	hockey puck
1 cup	baseball
2 cups	large grapefruit

RULE 3

EAT PROTEIN AT EVERY MEAL AND SNACK TO ELIMINATE CRAVINGS

Protein is an important part of the Skinny Gut Diet. You will eat protein at each meal and snack to help keep your appetite satisfied. Eating protein throughout the day will curb your cravings. Do you tend to crave snacks or sweets at mid-morning, mid-afternoon, or before bed? This is your body chasing the sugar high (and your unfriendly gut microbes chasing their next meal).

Proteins to Enjoy

Lean meats: Beef, chicken, turkey, buffalo, and lamb (organic is best, grass-fed when available)

Fish: Deep-water white fish, salmon, and sardines

Try to avoid fish high in mercury, such as mackerel, marlin, orange roughy, shark, swordfish, tilefish, and ahi and albacore tuna.

Eggs: Do not be afraid to eat eggs. Eggs are a simple source of protein that has been wrongly blamed for raising cholesterol. Fortunately, experts are changing their advice on egg consumption.

Nuts and seeds: Walnuts, almonds, pecans, macadamias, cashews, hazelnuts, pine nuts, and Brazil nuts, as well as flax, chia, pumpkin, sunflower, and sesame seeds. When possible, choose raw nuts.

It's helpful to soak raw almonds, cashews, and other nuts in water overnight to increase their digestibility. If you do so, refrigerate and eat within 24 hours or dehydrate and store.

Low-carb flours: Almond, coconut, and garbanzo flours are particularly useful for making delicious baked goods.

Dairy: If you do not have a dairy intolerance, sensitivity, or allergy, dairy is okay on the Skinny Gut Diet. Organic dairy is preferred. Some people best tolerate raw dairy, and others do well with goat- and sheep-derived dairy products.

Low-carb milks: Unsweetened nut milks, such as coconut milk and almond milk, soy milk (if you're not sensitive to soy), and hemp milk, are great dairy milk alternatives.

Tempeh: A fermented soybean food, tempeh doubles your benefit by packing the protein while also being a living food.

Tofu: Tofu is a good source of vegetable protein.

Hummus: Made of chickpeas and sesame paste, hummus is a

great snack option. Best if paired with deli meat or cheese for an extra protein boost. Be careful to not eat more than one serving at a time.

Meal-replacement shake: Protein shakes are a great way to get protein on the go. Plant-based shakes are excellent options.

With the exception of dairy, animal products—meat, fish, and eggs—do not contain carbohydrates. So you will not need to track your intake of these foods if you don't want to. However, be sure that you're eating protein at every meal and snack, so if you are keeping a food journal (more about that in Chapter 10), then simply record these foods so that you know you hit your target. For the other proteins, however—dairy, nuts and nut milks, tempeh, tofu, and hummus—you will need to track the teaspoons of sugar because they do contain some carbohydrates. Fortunately, these foods are usually packaged, so you can refer to the Nutrition Facts panel to apply my Teaspoon Tracker calculation.

How Much Protein?

You will be eating 12 portions of protein daily, at least. Again, protein is your ally when fighting cravings or hunger pangs. Eating protein at each meal and snack will help to keep your appetite satisfied.

Portion sizes are as follows:

Protein	Portion
Poultry, meat, seafood	1 ounce
Eggs	1 whole egg or 1 egg white
Tofu	3 ounces
Tempeh	1 ounce
Nuts	1 ounce (handful)
Nut butters	2 tablespoons
Plain Greek yogurt	3 ounces
Cheese	1 ounce

Tip: To incorporate protein snacks into your day, prepare then ahead of time and store them in small on-the-go containers for easy-to-grab snacks whenever you need them.

Breakfast: 2 portions
Lunch and Dinner: 3 to 4 portions
Snacks: 1 to 2 portions

Example:
A standard grilled chicken fillet added to a salad is 3 to 4 ounces, or 3 to 4 portions.

What About Beans?

You may have noticed that beans and lentils are not listed under protein. While legumes are a good source of protein, they are also high in carbohydrates as well as phytates—compounds that are difficult to digest. For these reasons, it is best to limit your bean consumption. However, in the STAY LEAN PHASE, you can eat legumes in moderation if they agree with you digestively. If you eat beans, be sure to soak them first to reduce the phytate content. Beans and legumes are higher in starchy carbohydrates, *so be sure to only eat one serving.*

Made of chickpeas and sesame paste, hummus is a great snack treat option and can be eaten *in moderation* during the GET LEAN PHASE. Hummus is best if paired with deli meat or cheese for an extra protein boost. Be careful *not to eat more than one serving at a time.* The carbs in hummus can really add up quickly. Remember to track your teaspoons of sugar.

What About Alcohol?

You may be wondering if you can drink alcohol on the Skinny Gut Diet. Rest assured, if you like to have a drink on occasion, you may. But you will have to limit your alcohol to wine or spirits. Beer is very high in carbohydrates as are many mixed drinks. You should steer clear of beer and sweetened juices and mixes, but you can enjoy an occasional glass of wine or spirit that is low in sugar. Eliminating alcohol is best, but not necessary.

Non-Alcoholic Beverages

Drink at least half your body weight in ounces of water daily; lemon or lime juice may be added

Herbal teas

Green tea

Sparkling or soda water

Vegetable juices (see drink recipes in Chapter 10)

Coffee or tea with natural, non-sugar sweeteners

Sweeteners

You will want to steer clear of artificial sweeteners (the pink, blue, or yellow packets) because they are not natural and have been linked to negative health effects. There are great natural alternatives that will sweeten your food and drinks without the added sugar.

Stevia

Lo han (also called monk fruit); see Resources (page 256) for recommended products

Sugar alcohols such as xylitol, erythritol, mannitol, and so on

Let's Put Some Meals and Snacks Together

Breakfast: For your breakfast protein, you might choose an egg cooked in coconut oil, some cheese, sausage or bacon, or even lox. In a hurry? A meal-replacement shake high in protein is a great option. To get some veggies in at breakfast, you might sauté some onions, spinach, and peppers and add them to your eggs, or eat them alongside sausage or bacon. You could also add berries to plain Greek yogurt. Or if you are in a hurry, add some berries and/or spinach and avocado to your meal-replacement shake, making a delicious shake.

> **Examples:**
> Veggie omelet
> Meal-replacement shake
> Plain Greek yogurt and berries

Lunch: Depending on your schedule, you may be bringing your lunch with you to work (plan ahead!), eating out, or preparing lunch at home. Lunch protein might be grilled chicken tenders (unbreaded) or a piece of salmon, egg salad, or even leftovers from the previous night's dinner. And if you are in a hurry, you can always have a meal-replacement shake for lunch. To get your veggies, you might eat a salad of mixed greens, or add a side of steamed or sautéed non-starchy vegetables to your lunch.

> **Examples:**
> Cobb salad
> Salmon with steamed broccoli
> Egg salad over mixed greens

Dinner: For your dinner protein, your imagination is the limit. Chicken, fish, meat, tofu, tempeh, and cheeses will be the mainstay of your dinner plate. Add plenty of nonstarchy veggies—steamed, sautéed, or raw as a salad—to your protein and you will have a well-balanced, delicious, and satisfying meal. Take your pick of your favorite nonstarchy veggies and season them with herbs, or dress your salad with extra-virgin olive oil and vinegar, or a vinaigrette (with no added sugar).

Examples:
Chicken breast with sautéed zucchini and onions, and a side
    salad of mixed greens
Slow Cooker Chicken Parmigiana (page 150)
More delicious dinner recipes in Chapter 13

Snacks: For snacks, your protein might be some slices of turkey or other deli meat, cheese, a small container of plain Greek yogurt, a handful of nuts and seeds, a serving of almond butter, or even a meal-replacement shake. To get your veggies at snack time, you could eat a leaf or two of lettuce with your deli meat, ¼ cup of berries with your yogurt, or a serving of celery with your almond butter.

Examples:
Turkey roll-up in a romaine leaf
Mini Cucumber "Sandwiches" (page 140)

Green drinks: A really great way to get your daily veggies is in a green drink. Most often enjoyed with a lunch or snack, the vibrant nutrients that green drinks provide are a sure-fire way to rejuvenate your day. A green drink is a vegetable juice that retains its fiber, and is made using a high-powered blender (see Resources, page 254, for my recommendations).

Example:
Celery, kale, apple, and lemon—refreshing! (See pages 144 to
    145 for recipes.)

Fermented Foods: On the Skinny Gut Diet you will add at least one serving of fermented foods daily with any meal or snack. I know that if I forget to eat my fermented food one day, I really miss it. I can almost feel it helping to balance my gut.

Examples:

Kefir in your meal-replacement shake

Sauerkraut as an addition to salads, meats, or cooked veggies—your choice; and please don't cook your kraut—you will kill the beneficial bacteria

> Not all sauerkraut is equal. The sauerkraut you buy from the grocery store is most likely pasteurized, and so it doesn't contain beneficial bacteria. See Resources, page 253, for my recommended products.

Timing Your Meals and Snacks

It's important to eat every two or three hours! After a few weeks, you will become sensitive to this schedule, as it becomes part of your daily routine. Honor the regular schedule to the best of your ability. If your daily schedule looks different from this, make the proper adjustments to the hours, as needed.

Time	Meal / Snack
7:00 A.M.	Breakfast
10:00 A.M.	Snack
12:00 P.M.	Lunch
3:00 P.M.	Snack
6:00 P.M.	Dinner
8:00 P.M.	Snack

Of course, your schedule may vary from time to time. You may have a snack at 6:00 P.M. and dinner at 8:00 P.M. because of a long work commute, as did one of the Skinny Gut Diet participants. That won't be a problem if you are prepared with snacks, no matter what your schedule. Do your best to avoid eating after 8:00 at night because this can impair your digestion and slow your weight loss. If possible, allow two to three hours after your last meal or snack before bedtime. And be sure your last snack contains protein.

MEAL		tsp sugar
7 A.M. Breakfast		**0.6**
Veggie scramble	2 eggs + ½ cup spinach + ¼ cup onion	
10 A.M. Snack		**1.7**
Meal-Replacement Shake (page 146)	Meal-Replacement Shake + ½ cup strawberries	
12:30 P.M. Lunch		**1.7**
Chicken salad over romaine with sauerkraut	3 oz. chicken + 1 tsp. mayo + ½ red bell pepper + 1 cup romaine + ½ cup sauerkraut	
3 P.M. Snack		**1.6**
2 celery stalks with almond butter	4 tbsp. almond butter + 2 celery stalks	
6 P.M. Dinner		**0.8**
Grilled salmon with steamed veggies	4 oz. salmon + ½ cup broccoli + ½ cup cauliflower	
8:00 P.M. Snack		**2.1**
Berries-n-Cream (page 223)	½ cup mixed berries + 1 container plain Greek yogurt + 4 tbsp. whipped cream	
TOTAL		**8.5**

In the Beginning

During the first couple weeks of the Skinny Gut Diet, your main adjustment will involve ridding yourself of the hold that carbohydrates have had over you. Yes, you will lose the carb cravings that come under the guise of a sweet tooth or the urge for crunchy, salty treats.

You know the feeling. It's 11:00 A.M. and lunch seems far on the horizon. You eat a cookie (or three) or chips to tide you over. Or maybe you are more the mid-afternoon snacker who needs a boost to get you over the afternoon slump. Or, you might be the type who considers a sweet treat after dinner to be an everyday occurrence.

These carbohydrate cravings have dragged us down for long enough. No more. I have designed the Skinny Gut Diet to help you minimize those cravings and rescue you from this vicious cycle. This is your long-awaited road to success.

As you begin, it may seem as though this program is all about protein. I mentioned protein in Chapter 7 and described it earlier here in this chapter, too. You may be wondering: *Why such a heavy focus on protein?* It's to halt your cravings. As I have said, and as you will discover for yourself, when you eat protein every two to three hours, your carb cravings will diminish 100 percent of the time.

I am not saying that you need to eat a large steak, half a chicken, or a block of tofu every couple hours. The beauty of protein is that even a 1- or 2-ounce serving of protein is enough to satisfy your appetite and keep those cravings at bay. *The key is regularity.* When someone from my program came to me saying that the diet wasn't "working," I reviewed the participant's food journal and found that she had forgotten to eat protein every two to three hours. After we fixed that problem, the weight came off and the cravings disappeared.

What if I am a vegetarian?

The Skinny Gut Diet emphasizes proteins, many in the form of animal products. If you are lacto-vegetarian, or lacto-ovo vegetarian, you will be able to eat dairy and eggs to obtain enough protein. For vegans, however, it will be difficult to eat a diet low in teaspoons of sugar. Beans, although high in protein and fiber, are also high in carbohydrates. You would have a difficult time getting enough protein from beans, nuts, and seeds without exceeding your daily total of teaspoons of sugar. However, you will likely still benefit if you focus on obtaining your carbohydrates from nonstarchy vegetables and low-sugar fruits (rather than from grains and processed foods) while being sure to eat enough protein daily. If you are vegetarian because meat doesn't agree with you, digestively, your body may not be producing enough digestive enzymes. You may find that taking digestive enzymes with every meal and snack significantly decreases your inability to tolerate meat.

Always remember to stay within 8 to 10 teaspoons of sugar daily while in the GET LEAN PHASE.

$$\left(\begin{array}{c} \text{TOTAL} \\ \text{CARBOHYDRATES} \end{array} - \text{DIETARY FIBER} \right) \div 5 = \quad \begin{array}{c} \text{TEASPOONS} \\ \text{OF SUGAR} \end{array}$$

CHAPTER 9 SUMMARY

During the GET LEAN PHASE you will eat 8 to 10 teaspoons of sugar daily while following the three simple rules:

➤ Rule 1: Eat more fat (*healthy* fat) to reduce silent inflammation.
➤ Rule 2: Eat living foods every day to balance your gut.
➤ Rule 3: Eat protein at every meal and snack to eliminate cravings.

You will remain in the GET LEAN PHASE until you reach your ideal weight. Then, you will move to the STAY LEAN PHASE (see Chapter 12). Nice and simple—three steps, two phases, one skinny you.

Recap of foods to eliminate or reduce:

- All foods containing gluten or wheat. You will be surprised at what foods contain gluten or wheat. If you find that you are still having trouble losing weight even though you are following the diet to a tee, you may have a stronger sensitivity to gluten. See Resources, page 257, for testing that will help you better understand your sensitivity.
- All grains during the GET LEAN PHASE.
- Sugars and artificial sweeteners: sugar, honey, fructose, molasses, maple syrup, corn syrup, agave syrup, and any foods containing these.
- Most fruits other than those mentioned previously.
- All fruit juices unless greatly diluted.
- Breads, rolls, crackers, cookies, and cakes unless made from grain-free flours such as almond or coconut flour.
- Alcohol: limit alcohol to twice weekly, one glass of wine or spirits. Eliminating alcohol is best, but limited intake is okay if this is your preference. Wine will add to your daily sugar, as each glass of wine is approximately 1 teaspoon sugar.

Chapter 10

POWER TOOLS

In my years of refining the Skinny Gut Diet, I realized that certain tools are helpful to ensure success. I call these "power tools," and I made sure that the participants of the Skinny Gut Diet program had access to them all. Now I share them with you.

POWER TOOL #1: LUNCHBOX AND FOOD CONTAINERS

Organizing your snacks and meals is the key to reaching your goal of having a skinny gut. A dedicated lunchbox with small containers that nest inside will make your preparations easier. Personally, I like to use a small Igloo Playmate lunch cooler. It has a pocket for an icepack and easily holds a 3-cup Pyrex flat, rectangular container (for your lunch) along with two 1-cup round containers (for your snacks). These three pieces make one set.

Be sure to get at least two sets so that one is always handy when you need it. You can even prepare two or three lunches at a time to get ready for your week. You can fit a small container of yogurt into the top area of the lunchbox, and a handful of nuts or your favorite Skinny Gut snack in a baggie, just in case. You'll be set for your day. I usually prepare my food the night before so that I can load my lunchbox and dash off to work.

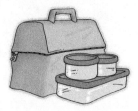

"The lunchbox and food containers power tool was my favorite. It helped me to prepare lunch in 'measures,' which helped me to not overeat." —Cynthia

My husband, Stan, is one of the early success stories of the Skinny Gut Diet. Years later, he is still as excited as he was when he lost those 40 pounds. He asked me to tell you how sharp your awareness will become of when it's time to eat (remember, every two to three hours) and how you will come to prefer eating a protein snack rather than a high-carb one.

When Stan had started on this eating plan, he used to stuff the containers as full as he possibly could with protein. Yes, those containers were bursting. They hold roughly 2 ounces, but Stan, previously a "volume eater," wanted to get as much bang for the buck as he could. He pushed those 2 ounces toward 3 or 4 ounces. That was okay, though, because protein was his ally. Today, Stan fills those containers half full, if that. Once he reached his balanced weight, his desire to overeat became a distant memory.

This change in outlook happened for all of the Skinny Gut participants, and it will happen for you, too. Stan wants you to hear this loud and clear: the Skinny Gut Diet really works.

POWER TOOL #2: SNACKS

Although snacking is sometimes thought of as a bad habit, if you think about it, that's because most snacks are filled with carbs and sugar. You crave these foods because they stimulate you as they spike your blood sugar. When it drops, you crave more carbs for another spike. To break this vicious cycle, in the Skinny Gut Diet you will be eating frequently—snacks are absolutely necessary. Your snacks will always contain protein (at least 1 to 2 ounces), which will douse your carb cravings and help mold your skinny gut.

Stan's favorite snack was quite a hit with the Skinny Gut Diet participants. He prepares what we call "roll-ups." In fact, we don't leave home without them. To make Stan's roll-up, you simply layer a slice of deli meat, a slice of cheese, and a leaf of lettuce and roll it up. Wrap in a paper towel or wax paper and place three roll-ups in a baggie. They fit perfectly into the lunchbox. No matter where we go, there they are. Just peel back the paper and enjoy. (I have to fight my Cavalier Springer Spaniels for them!)

The Skinny Gut Diet motto: Be prepared.

Don't find yourself without a snack handy. Alexandra, one of the Skinny Gut Diet participants, left her house unprepared one day. She thought she would be able to find something to eat at the hospital where she was training. She didn't get a break to grab some food, and by the time she was able to find a moment to herself, the only things available were the high-carb snacks from the vending machine. She did not succumb, but did feel hungry and had developed a headache. She vowed to never leave home unprepared again.

Skinny Gut Snack Ideas

Apple and Nut Butter
½ Granny Smith apple + 1 tablespoon almond butter =
2 teaspoons sugar

Blackberries and Cottage Cheese
4 ounces cottage cheese + ½ cup blackberries =
1.3 teaspoons sugar

Celery and Roasted Red Pepper Hummus
2 ribs celery + 2 tablespoons Roasted Red Pepper Hummus
(page 142) = 1.5 teaspoons sugar

Baby Carrots and Hummus
½ cup baby carrots + ½ cup hummus = 2 teaspoons sugar

Smoked Salmon and Celery
Shredded smoked salmon + 1 teaspoon mayo + black pepper
+ 2 ribs celery = 0 teaspoons sugar

Handful of Nuts (prepare a few portions of nuts to grab on the go)
¼ cup mixed nuts (without peanuts) = 1.2 teaspoons sugar

Handful of Almonds
20 almonds = ½ teaspoon sugar

Roast Beef and Asparagus Roll-up
1 slice roast beef + 1 tablespoon cream cheese + 2 asparagus
spears = 0.6 teaspoons sugar

Mini Cucumber "Sandwiches"
6 slices cucumber + 3 squares of Cheddar cheese + 1 slice turkey
breast = 0.1 teaspoons sugar

Cucumber Canoes
½ cucumber sliced in half lengthwise and hollowed out +
1 ounce cottage cheese + 1 teaspoon fresh dill =
1.1 teaspoons sugar

Zucchini Chips
2 cups ultra-thin-sliced zucchini (use a mandoline) +
½ teaspoon olive oil + salt and pepper + 135°F dehydrator or
oven for 5 to 6 hours = 0.6 teaspoons sugar

Sauerkraut and Seeds
½ cup sauerkraut + ¼ cup roasted pumpkin seeds =
1.5 teaspoons sugar

Plain Greek Yogurt

6-ounce container of yogurt = 1.7 teaspoons of sugar (add berries
and chia seeds when you have a hankering for sweets)

Whipped Cream Sundae

¼ cup whipped cream + ¼ cup berries + handful of nuts =
1.4 teaspoons sugar

TURKEY-GUAC ROLL-UPS

0.4 teaspoon sugar
10 minutes to prepare
Serves 3

3 large ripe Hass avocados
½ red onion, chopped
2 garlic cloves, minced
1 teaspoon ground cumin
2 small limes, juiced
2 tablespoons chopped fresh cilantro
4 scallions, green and white parts thinly sliced
15 deli turkey slices

1. Cut the avocados in half and remove the seeds. Scoop out and
mash the flesh well in a bowl.

2. Combine all the other ingredients except the turkey and mix
well. Spread the guacamole on deli turkey slices. Roll up and eat as a
snack.

TURKEY-HUMMUS ROLL-UPS

1.2 teaspoons sugar
5 minutes to prepare
Serves 1

6 tablespoons Roasted Red Pepper Hummus (recipe follows)
3 thick slices deli turkey
Lettuce leaves

Spread 2 tablespoons of the hummus on each turkey slice. Lay the turkey slice on a lettuce leaf. Roll up and enjoy.

Roasted Red Pepper Hummus
(in moderation)
1.5 teaspoons sugar
15 minutes to prepare
Serves 30

> One 7-ounce jar roasted red peppers, rinsed and drained
> One 15-ounce can chickpeas, rinsed and drained
> One 15-ounce can cannellini beans, rinsed and drained
> ¼ cup tahini
> 3 garlic cloves
> 2 tablespoons fresh lemon juice
> 1 teaspoon ground cumin
> 2 tablespoons plain Greek yogurt
> Salt and freshly ground black pepper

Add all the ingredients except the salt and pepper to a food processor. Process until mixture is smooth. Season with salt and pepper. Chill for at least 30 minutes and serve.

POWER TOOL #3: DIGITAL KITCHEN FOOD SCALE

For at least the first week or two when you're on the Skinny Gut Diet, it will be very helpful to measure the amounts of your food so that you get to know, visually, how much 3 ounces of protein is or how many nuts equal 1 ounce. I made sure that every one of the Skinny Gut Diet participants had a scale, which turned out to be really useful as we designed and shared recipes with each other. If you know the proper weights of your foods, you will be able to better figure out the teaspoons of sugar in any recipe. This power tool is not absolutely necessary, but you will likely find it helpful.

POWER TOOL #4: BLENDER AND SHAKER CUP

You can find wonderful power-packed blenders on the market these days that do more than blend a simple shake. They turn vegetables and fruits into blended drinks that help you get plenty of nutrients without losing the fiber; standard juicers strain out the fiber. You can blend green drinks (recipes follow), meal-replacement shakes, salad dressings, sauces, and dips all with the push of a button or the turn of a dial. See Resources, page 254, for my recommendations.

Let's face it, no matter how healthy you are, you are still probably challenged to get enough veggies into your diet. After a few weeks on the Skinny Gut Diet, I saw that some participants were not eating the five to nine daily servings of fruits and vegetables I had recommended. To solve this problem, I made sure everyone had a blender.

"We love the power tools. They made preparing food so much more fun! We use the Ninja blender and our Crock-Pot often to make life easier." —Sandi and Dave

I share with you here some of the green drink recipes that helped the Skinny Gut Diet participants get their greens while also pleasing their palate with low-sugar fruits. The participants ranged from fast-food frequenters to health-food store shoppers, yet all of them found green drinks that they enjoyed. Adding milk kefir to the drinks supplemented the protein and fermented foods while making a creamy mix; spinning in some nut butters also added protein. Using spinach and lettuce doesn't call for a big shift in taste, but kale and parsley will have a greater impact on flavor. Experiment according to your own tastes. Be mindful of the amount of apples, carrots, and beets that you add, because these foods can raise your sugar measures if you are not careful. Adding a natural sweetener like stevia or lo han (monk fruit) will help, if you prefer a sweeter blend.

GREEN JUICE

2.9 teaspoons sugar
10 minutes to prepare
Serves 1

⅓ small cucumber
2 ribs celery
1 cup trimmed kale
1 cup baby spinach
3 sprigs parsley
Juice from 1 lemon wedge
¼ Granny Smith apple

Place ingredients in Ninja or Vitamix and blend until smooth. Enjoy.

REFRESHING JUICE

2.7 teaspoons sugar
10 minutes to prepare
Serves 1

4 ribs celery
1 cup trimmed kale
⅓ lemon
¼ Granny Smith apple

Place ingredients in Ninja or Vitamix and blend until smooth. Enjoy.

HAPPY DIGESTION JUICE

1 teaspoon sugar
10 minutes to prepare
Serves 1

2 ribs celery
1 cup chopped green cabbage
⅓ lemon

Place ingredients in Ninja or Vitamix and blend until smooth. Enjoy.

MINERALS WITH A ZING JUICE

3 teaspoons sugar
10 minutes to prepare
Serves 1

½ cup trimmed kale
½ carrot
¼ cucumber
½ rib celery
¼ Granny Smith apple
⅓ lemon

Place ingredients in Ninja or Vitamix and blend until smooth. Enjoy.

I have always been a big fan of meal-replacement shakes for those of us who are on the go, juggling jobs and responsibilities, but still intent on getting proper nutrition each day. In the Skinny Gut Diet group, participants used meal-replacement shakes for different reasons. Sometimes they needed a quick and easy breakfast or lunch, and other times they grabbed it as an emergency snack. The group enjoyed both chocolate and vanilla shakes as a regular part of their eating plans.

Here is one basic recipe that can be prepared in a blender or can be combined in a shaker cup without the fruit. If you are not familiar with shaker cups, these are simply cups with lids that also have a stainless steel wire ball inside that helps to mix the drink when you shake the cup. It's a great way to mix up a meal-replacement shake when you are on the go.

MEAL-REPLACEMENT SHAKE

Serves 1

1 serving meal-replacement supplement powder

1 cup unsweetened almond milk

½ cup frozen berries (optional)

Place ingredients in a blender (with fruit) or shaker cup (without fruit), and blend (or shake) until smooth. Enjoy.

POWER TOOL #5: SLOW COOKER

Everyone in the Skinny Gut Diet group, without exception, was busy, so I wanted to provide the best tools that would help them nourish their bodies and simplify their preparations. Personally, I use my slow cooker on a regular basis—at least a couple times a week. It is an easy way to prepare meals for my family while I am at work. Stan and I also like to use the leftovers for lunches and snacks. I toss a few ingredients into the pot, set the cooking level and time, and eight hours later, I come home to something fantastic.

> **"I had a slow cooker, but it had been hidden in my pantry. Now I use it regularly." —Danielle**

Slow cookers are also a great way to prepare your own meats for snacks. It's so easy to cook a boneless turkey breast in the cooker and thinly slice it to make homemade deli turkey. Each week I made a different slow cooker meal for the group. I hope you will enjoy the simple recipes that I am sharing with you here. These slow cooker recipes are in addition to the breakfast, lunch, dinner, snacks, and "sweets" recipes found on pages 180 to 226.

SLOW COOKER PORK RIBS

0.8 teaspoon sugar
10 minutes to prepare, 8 hours to cook
Serves 8

3 pounds baby back pork ribs, with membrane removed
Stubb's Beef Marinade
Lysander's Pork Rub

1. Coat the ribs with the pork rub.

2. Cut between the ribs into single pieces and place in the slow cooker. Pour the marinade over the ribs.

3. Cover and cook on low heat for 8 hours. Serve with Spicy Sautéed Kale (page 222).

SLOW COOKER CHUCK ROAST

0.4 teaspoons of sugar
10 minutes to prepare, 8 hours to cook
Serves 12

3 pound boneless chuck roast
Grill Mates Montreal Seasoning (or another brand of seasoning)
1 cup chicken stock
1 tablespoon minced garlic
1 onion, chopped
One 14-ounce can diced tomatoes

1. Coat the roast with the seasoning. Pour the stock into the slow cooker. Add the roast.

2. Combine the garlic, onion, and tomatoes and pour over meat. Cover and cook on low heat for 8 hours.

SLOW COOKER BEEF STEW

2 teaspoons sugar
30 minutes to prepare, 8 hours to cook
Serves 8

2 pounds boneless beef sirloin, cubed
One 14-ounce can stewed tomatoes
One 14-ounce can spicy fire-roasted tomatoes
1 onion, chopped
1 tablespoon minced garlic
2 bay leaves
2 cups beef stock
1 pound carrots, sliced
8 ounces frozen or fresh green beans

1. Place the beef in the slow cooker. Cover with both tomatoes, the onion, garlic, bay leaves, and stock. Cover and cook on low heat for 6 hours.

2. Add the carrots and green beans, cover, and cook for 2 more hours on low heat. Remove the bay leaves before serving.

SLOW COOKER PORK TENDERLOIN

0.4 teaspoon sugar
15 minutes to prepare, 8 hours to cook
Serves 8

2 pound boneless pork tenderloin
Lysander's Pork Rub (or another brand of pork rub)
½ Granny Smith apple
1 tablespoon garlic, minced
1 medium onion, chopped

1. Rub the pork sparingly with the rub. Place in the slow cooker.

2. Add the apple, garlic, and onion, then cover and cook on low heat for 8 hours.

SLOW COOKER CHICKEN CACCIATORE

1.5 teaspoons sugar

30 minutes to prepare, 7 to 9 hours to cook

Serves 12

1 teaspoon onion powder

1 teaspoon garlic powder

1 teaspoon dried oregano

1 teaspoon dried basil

¾ teaspoon freshly ground black pepper

6 boneless, skinless chicken breast halves

3 boneless, skinless chicken thighs, cut in half

1 tablespoon coconut oil

2 cups sliced button mushrooms

1½ cups sliced red bell peppers

1½ cups sliced green bell peppers

1 cup thinly sliced onion

One 28-ounce can tomatoes

One 6-ounce can tomato paste

2 bay leaves

1 tablespoon balsamic vinegar

1. Mix the dried seasonings and dredge the chicken breasts and thighs in the spices. Set aside.

2. Put 1 tablespoon coconut oil in the bottom of the slow cooker. Add the mushrooms, peppers, and onion. Add the tomatoes, tomato paste, bay leaves, and vinegar. Layer on the spiced chicken and any remaining spices.

3. Cover and cook on low heat for 7 to 9 hours. Remove the bay leaves and serve.

SLOW COOKER CHICKEN PARMIGIANA

1.3 teaspoons sugar
30 minutes to prepare, 6 to 7 (or 3 to 4) hours to cook
Serves 8

   1 tablespoon olive oil
   ½ cup gluten-free bread crumbs
   ¼ cup grated Parmesan cheese
   ¼ teaspoon dried oregano
   ¼ teaspoon dried basil
   ¼ teaspoon freshly ground black pepper
   ¼ teaspoon salt
   Pinch of red pepper flakes (optional)
   1 large egg
   4 boneless, skinless chicken breast halves
   3 ounces mozzarella cheese, sliced or grated
   One 24-ounce jar marinara sauce (no added sugar)

1. Coat the bottom of a slow cooker with olive oil.

2. Mix the bread crumbs, Parmesan cheese, and spices in a medium bowl. Beat the egg in a second bowl. Dip each chicken breast into the egg and then into the spice mixture, coating both sides of the chicken with the crumbs. Place each breast in the slow cooker.

3. Cover the chicken with the mozzarella cheese, then pour the marinara sauce over and cover. Cook on low heat for 6 to 7 hours (or on high heat for 3 to 4 hours).

4. Serve over Spaghetti Squash "Pasta" (page 221), julienned raw (or lightly sautéed) zucchini, or cooked and drained low-carb pasta (see Resources, page 254).

SLOW COOKER MEAT SAUCE

0.8 teaspoon sugar
30 minutes to prepare, 8 hours to cook
Serves 12

2 tablespoons olive oil

1 onion, chopped

1 tablespoon minced garlic

2 pounds ground turkey

4 large links mild Italian-flavored chicken sausage

One 24-ounce jar tomato sauce (no added sugar)

One 14-ounce can crushed fire-roasted tomatoes

1. Heat the olive oil in a medium sauté pan. Sauté the onion and garlic until soft, about 5 minutes. Add the ground turkey and sauté until browned, about 8 minutes. Place the mixture in the slow cooker.

2. Slice the chicken sausage and add to the sauté pan, sautéing until browned, about 8 minutes.

3. Add the sausage to the slow cooker, then add the tomato sauce and crushed tomatoes. Cover and cook on low heat for 8 hours.

4. Serve over Spaghetti Squash "Pasta" (page 221), julienned raw (or lightly sautéed) zucchini, or cooked and drained low-carb pasta (see Resources, page 254).

ZESTY LEMON HERB TURKEY BREAST, SLOW COOKER STYLE

0.4 teaspoon sugar
30 minutes to prepare, 4 to 5 hours to cook
Serves 8

Juice and zest of 2 lemons

2 tablespoons minced fresh rosemary

1 teaspoon crumbled dried sage

2 tablespoons Dijon mustard

½ cup water

2 garlic cloves, crushed

Salt and freshly ground black pepper

1 turkey London broil, about 2 pounds

1. Mix all the ingredients except the turkey to make the marinade.

2. Place the turkey in a bowl, pour in the marinade, and turn the breast to coat well. Marinate, refrigerated, for 4 to 6 hours or overnight.

3. Place the turkey and marinade in the slow cooker. Cover and cook on low heat for 8 hours or until tender.

4. Serve with vegetables or salad, or thinly slice to eat as a homemade deli meat.

POWER TOOL #6: DAILY FOOD JOURNAL

To gain a good idea about how to eat on the Skinny Gut Diet, keep a daily food journal, at least in the beginning. I used two different styles of journals—one on paper and one electronic. Choose what works best for you.

You will need to keep track of your teaspoons of sugar, using my Teaspoon Tracker, but I also recommend that you keep track of your daily servings of nonstarchy vegetables and low-sugar fruits, as a way to ensure you are eating at least five servings of these daily. Simply record your foods and use the Teaspoon Tracker to determine the sugar totals in the foods you are eating. For vegetables and fruits, refer to the charts on pages 123 to 125. For prepared foods that do not have labels, you can break down the composition by looking up the nutrition facts online or in reference materials (see my recommendations on page 255).

$$\left(\begin{array}{c} \text{TOTAL} \\ \text{CARBOHYDRATES} \end{array} - \text{DIETARY FIBER} \right) \div 5 = \quad \begin{array}{c} \text{TEASPOONS} \\ \text{OF SUGAR} \end{array}$$

If you prefer to go the electronic route, which is easier for calculating the teaspoons of sugar in prepared foods, check out the website and app My Fitness Pal. This site offers a huge diversity of foods and brands, and it makes tracking your meals easy. It will give you your total carbohydrates and fiber (along with many other nutrients) for each meal and for the entire day. Simply plug the carbohydrate and dietary fiber totals into the Teaspoon Tracker calculation and you will have your total teaspoons of sugar. Our group used both paper tracking and electronic tracking at first, but by the end everyone was using My Fitness Pal. It was more convenient for them, but you can decide what works best for you.

After you have tracked your sugar totals for about a month, you will have a good idea of how to create that skinny gut. You may want to continue recording your meals as a way to stay on track, especially until you reach your Skinny Gut goal. A food journal is a great tool when you're starting out, especially if you are the type who likes to monitor your progress. Later on, if you find yourself reverting to old ways, use your food journal again, and you will be back into the swing of things in no time.

POWER TOOL #7: BATHROOM SCALE

Across the board, people have a desire for two things: to look good and to feel good. When you balance your gut with the Skinny Gut Diet suggestions, your body will naturally achieve its healthy weight for your frame, and you'll feel great. On a practical level, we all like to see our numbers change, whether they are our weight, our pant size, or our waist measurement.

I recommend that you weigh yourself at regular intervals. Tracking your weight at home with a bathroom scale will be a great motivator. And let's face it, if you weigh yourself in the morning without clothes and after you have gone to the bathroom (ahem), you will be at your lowest weight.

POWER TOOL #8: SHARE THE SKINNY GUT DIET WITH OTHERS

Shifting your habits is never easy, no matter how clear your goals or simple your plans. We all know this. In fact, that's why you're reading this book: you want some help along the way. Looking back, I realize that perhaps the tool that has most helped me, as well as many others, to maintain our resolve is *sharing the journey with others*. The support that I have had—and given—over the years, and most recently with the Skinny Gut Diet participants, has been invaluable.

"From what I have learned on the Skinny Gut Diet, I am working not only with my husband but also with my grandmother and some friends. I hope we are all able to pay it forward." —Danielle

One married couple in our group, Sandi and Dave, created their skinny guts together. Two best friends, Alexandra and Danielle, challenged each other constantly. Cynthia and her mother learned together while her mother visited. They all mentioned frequently how helpful it was to have someone close by to support them in their new food choices. You may remember that Danielle's husband ended up losing 25 pounds after learning from Danielle. And Cynthia's mother lost 14 pounds after just a month of incorporating some of the Skinny Gut Diet concepts.

My assistant and I provided phone and e-mail support along the way, with nearly weekly meetings that were assisted by my sister Sandee. Through My Fitness Pal, many of the participants became "friends" with others and could message and support each other to help stay on track and share recipes and meal plans.

I want to be there for you, too. Visit skinnygutdiet.com, where you can access more tools and obtain more information, as well as interact with members of this community and support forum. They will help you reach your skinny gut goals. I look forward to seeing you there.

CHAPTER 10 SUMMARY

In my years of refining the Skinny Gut Diet, I realized that these power tools are very helpful to ensure success:

- ➤ Power Tool #1: Lunchbox and Food Containers
- ➤ Power Tool #2: Snacks
- ➤ Power Tool #3: Digital Kitchen Food Scale
- ➤ Power Tool #4: Blender and Shaker Cup
- ➤ Power Tool #5: Slow Cooker
- ➤ Power Tool #6: Daily Food Journal
- ➤ Power Tool #7: Bathroom Scale
- ➤ Power Tool #8: Share the Skinny Gut Diet with Others

Chapter 11

SKINNY GUT SUPPLEMENTS

Although I always say diet is 80 percent of the game, there are certain supplements that are critical to helping you achieve gut balance and weight loss. Your digestive health is the foundation for your overall health. Because of this, achieving optimal digestion is the first step toward reaching your ideal weight. There are four main supplements I recommend be taken daily by anyone with a digestive tract. I call this the H.O.P.E. Formula.

H.O.P.E. Formula
H is for High Fiber
O is for Omega-3
P is for Probiotics
E is for Enzymes

The H.O.P.E. Formula is a daily regimen that optimizes your digestive health. Following the H.O.P.E. Formula, you will balance your gut bacteria; you'll attain regular, satisfying bowel movements, and reduce the inflammation in your digestive tract; you'll put an end to digestive upsets and embarrassing symptoms like gas and bloating; and you'll fully digest your food and absorb the vital nutrients your body needs. This formula is a crucial part of the Skinny Gut Diet. A healthy diet and supplementation go hand in hand. Healthy foods will provide the bulk of your nutrition while supplements will help fill in the gaps. At the very minimum, you need to be taking probiotics and fiber while on the Skinny Gut Diet so that you can achieve optimal gut balance. Probiotics and fiber are an integral piece of the puzzle.

H is for High Fiber

As you are learning, fiber is one of the secrets to long-term weight loss and optimal digestive health and regularity. When you eat a high-fiber meal, you will feel satisfied rather than be reaching for the dessert menu.

There are four main ways that fiber helps you lose weight:

- Fiber helps promote gut balance by supporting the amounts of beneficial bacteria in your gut. When your gut is in balance, you can achieve your perfect weight for your body type.
- Fiber suppresses your appetite by stimulating the hormone cholecystokinin (CCK), which tells your brain to stop eating.
- Fiber eliminates extra calories from the food you eat through the fiber flush effect (fecal energy extraction).
- Fiber slows your body's conversion of carbohydrate to sugar, and so it supports blood sugar stability and helps you lose weight.

There are actually two types of fiber—soluble and insoluble—and all plant-based foods contain both, in varying ratios. You can think of fiber as a sponge. Soluble fiber is like the soft yellow side, soaking up unwanted toxins (as well as cholesterol) as it moves through the digestive tract. Soluble fiber is the type that feeds the good bacteria in your gut—it's the prebiotic. Insoluble fiber is like the green scrubber side of the sponge, helping to sweep the colon free of debris. Insoluble fiber provides bulk to the stool to promote regular, healthy bowel movements. Soluble fiber dissolves in water and leaves the stomach slowly, helping to control appetite and blood sugar levels. Insoluble fiber does not dissolve in water and travels through the intestine in much the same form as it was consumed. Foods high in soluble fiber are primarily fruits and vegetables. Foods high in insoluble fiber tend to be cereal grains (which you won't be eating), nuts, and seeds.

> "Before the Skinny Gut Diet I had bad stomach pains on a frequent basis. Since starting the program I have not had those pains anymore. I was never a person who would religiously take supplements, but this program changed my point of view. In a sense I feel naked without my H.O.P.E. formula." —Danielle

In Chapter 2, I discussed the effects of fiber on calorie absorption and appetite. I explained how fiber helps soak up extra calories and move them out of the body so that you won't absorb them. The fiber flush effect is responsible for subtracting calories from your diet. Think of fiber as a calorie escort, shuffling calories out of the body before they are absorbed.

You also learned that fiber triggers the hormone CCK, which sends a signal to your brain that tells you that you are no longer hungry. Among the first scientists to discover the effects of CCK was a team of researchers from the University of California at Davis. They found that women who ate a high-fiber meal released more CCK into their bloodstream than women who ate a low-fiber meal. The same was true of those who ate a high-fat meal as opposed to a low-fat meal.

Have you ever noticed that when you eat a lot of fat, as in a big juicy steak, you feel satisfied? Well, fat releases the same hormone, CCK. Those who ate the high-fat and high-fiber meals reported a greater feeling of fullness, which was attributed to higher levels of CCK in their bodies.

Fiber's stabilizing effects on blood sugar are also important to weight loss. If you overindulge in sugar or starchy carbohydrates at a meal, your blood sugar level will rise sharply, but it will soon fall back. When this happens, you usually experience a craving for more carbohydrates to bring your blood sugar back up (offsetting the feelings of shakiness, fatigue, brain fog, and dizziness that go with low blood sugar, or hypoglycemia). Habitual overconsumption of carbo-hydrates sets off a repetitive pattern of quick rises and drops in blood sugar levels. The good news is that fiber helps to slow the conversion of carbohydrates, so it can reverse blood sugar's roller-coaster rise and fall. Fiber helps normalize your blood sugar level, which calms any cravings.

> Try taking one serving of a fiber supplement before you eat and you'll find that you're not as hungry as you thought.

The best sources of fiber are fruits, vegetables, nuts, and seeds. Fibers are actually the nondigestible parts of plants, and they are found only in plant foods. Fiber is a critical element of good gut health, but the average American eats only between 10 and 15 grams per day, less than half of the suggested 20 to 35 grams. I recommend at least 35 grams of fiber daily, which is on the higher end of conventional recommendations. With 35 grams of fiber daily—from your diet and supplements—your digestive tract will get what it needs to function properly. I do recommend that you get a large portion of your fiber from nonstarchy vegetables and low-sugar fruits, but it can be diffi-cult to eat 35 grams of fiber from diet alone. A fiber supplement is an easy way to help you reach that daily goal.

When adding a fiber supplement to your daily regimen, you will want to start off slowly. Begin with one serving once daily for three days, and notice how you respond digestively. If you find that you are gassy, take half a serving daily until your digestive system adapts. Then you can go back up to one serving once daily, eventually work-ing up to as much as three servings a day.

What to look for in a fiber supplement:

- Find a fiber made with natural and organically grown ingre-dients.
- Look for organic acacia fiber or non-GMO corn fiber. If you prefer a great-tasting fruity fiber, look for a fruit fiber with

organic acacia or non-GMO corn fiber. The Skinny Gut Diet
participants used these fibers in the program.

- Other good sources of fiber are flax seeds and natural chia
  seeds.
- Choose a psyllium-free fiber to prevent cramping, gas, or
  bloating.
- A powdered fiber supplement is best to ensure that you are
  taking enough fiber.
- See Resources, page 255, for my product recommendations.

Dosage:

Take a fiber supplement in the morning and at night, along with
a glass of water. The fiber supplement can also be taken before
meals to reduce hunger.

O is for Omega-3

In 2009, the Harvard School of Public Health published a report
on the top preventable causes of death.[1] Most of them are what you
would expect—obesity and smoking, for example—but what's really
interesting is that no. 8 on the list was *not enough omega-3 fats*! According to the study, low dietary omega-3 intake is responsible for
84,000 deaths each year. These vital fats are missing in many Ameri-
cans' diets, a lack that is drastically affecting their health.

More than 11,000 reports, including 1,500 human clinical tri-
als, have been published on the benefits of fish oil and omega-3 fatty
acids. Omega-3s are one of the most well-studied nutrients and have
been found to be beneficial for a wide range of health conditions.
Omega-3s significantly improve cardiovascular, brain, joint, and digestive health, to name just a few benefits.

Although omega-3 fats don't directly affect weight gain, they do
play a crucial part in preventing and reversing silent inflammation
and in healing a leaky gut. Silent inflammation is the root cause of
most chronic diseases, and it plays a major role in weight gain, as you

have learned. It can be difficult to get enough omega-3 fats from diet alone unless you eat large portions of fish like salmon and sardines every single day. Taking a daily omega-3 fish oil supplement is a convenient way to optimize your omega-3 levels, balance your omega-3/6 ratio, and reduce silent inflammation.

"My mind, body, and soul feel like they have been renewed. I have been enjoying every minute of the new me." —Danielle

The diet humans today evolved from (the hunter-gatherer diet) consisted of almost equal portions of omega-3 and omega-6 fatty acids. Today's Standard American Diet (SAD), on the other hand, contains ten to twenty-five times the amount of omega-6s as opposed to omega-3s. That means we are eating a lot less omega-3 fats and a lot more omega-6 fats than our ancestors, a pattern that promotes the development of many diseases rooted in inflammation, including obesity. The SAD diet is overabundant in omega-6 fats, and is considered deficient in omega-3 fats.

The best way to obtain the benefits of omega-3s while avoiding the toxic contaminants they often contain—such as mercury, PCBs, and dioxins—is to consume a purified fish oil supplement. Not all fish oil supplements are without toxins, however, so be sure to read the label. Look for the International Fish Oil Standards (IFOS) icon on the bottle to be sure you are getting a purified, high-quality fish oil.

What to look for in a fish oil supplement:

- Purity: Look for the IFOS (International Fish Oil Standards) seal to ensure you are getting a high-quality, purified fish oil supplement.
- Potency: Look for a concentrated fish oil that contains at least 1,000 milligrams total omega-3 per softgel.
- Enteric-coated, dark-colored softgels: Look for an enteric-coated fish oil to minimize fishy repeat (belching);

dark-colored softgels help protect the oils from damaging light.
- Added lipase: Look for a fish oil supplement with added lipase, a fat-digesting enzyme that helps to improve the breakdown and absorption of omega-3 fats.
- See Resources, page 255, for my product recommendations.

Dosage:

Take at least 2,000 mg of total omega-3 daily. (Be sure that you are taking 2,000 mg of omega-3 and not just 2,000 mg of fish oil.)

What to Look for in an Omega-3 Fish Oil Supplement:

	Amount per Fish Gel
Vitamin D3 (cholecalciferol)	1,000 IU
Total Omega 3•5•6•7•9•11	1,100 mg
Omega-3	1,025 mg
EPA (Eicosapentaenoic Acid)	780 mg
DHA (Docosahexaenoic Acid)	120 mg
Omega-5	1 mg
Omega-6	56 mg
Omega-7	1 mg
Omega-9	12 mg
Omega-11	1 mg
Lipase (activity 50 FIP)	5 mg

P is for Probiotics

By now you know that gut bacteria and probiotics are your inner secrets to weight loss. On the Skinny Gut Diet you are eating foods that feed the good bacteria and starve the bad bacteria. Sadly, you may have started with a gut imbalance that likely began during childhood, which means it will require continual replenishment to maintain a beneficial balance of gut bacteria. Taking a probiotic supplement each day will help ensure you are adding enough good bacteria to make a difference. After all, your gut contains 100 trillion bacteria, so you will want the high-potency probiotic supplement to have an impact on your health.

Probiotics are the friendly gut bacteria that serve as our body's own gut protection system (GPS). Your GPS works in three main ways:

1. It produces substances that neutralize harmful bacteria.
2. It protects the intestinal lining and improves the balance of good-to-bad bacteria in the gut by crowding out bad bacteria.
3. It influences the immune system so that it responds appropriately to invaders, such as harmful organisms, toxins, and even food.

Good bacteria have been part of the human diet for thousands of years, largely in the form of fermented foods. In 1906, Russian scientist Elie Metchnikoff proposed the concept of the probiotic "Bulgarian bacillus," now known as *Lactobacillus bulgaricus*. Metchnikoff is known as the Grandfather of Probiotics. He attributed the long life spans of Bulgarians to the fermented milk they drank. He isolated the *Lactobacillus* bacteria in this milk and proposed that he could introduce this bacteria to the guts of people not drinking fermented milk, producing a beneficial change in gut bacterial balance. Metchnikoff's studies led to more research on the effects of bacteria on intestinal health, eventually resulting in the availability of probiotic products that addressed digestive disruptions.

Research on probiotics has increased dramatically during the past few decades. It is now recognized that individual probiotic strains have unique qualities. One strain may have specific immune-boosting properties while another may offer stronger ability to resist pathogens in the gut. For these reasons, and because of the wide diversity of bacteria that exist in the gut, a multistrain probiotic formula that closely resembles the diversity of a healthy gut may be more beneficial than a single-strain formula.[2]

Probiotics can be obtained through the diet by eating yogurt, kefir, and certain other fermented foods (all part of the Skinny Gut Diet), but at times these products do not contain high amounts of probiotics. In addition, fermented foods contain *Lactobacillus* probiotics but are lacking in Bifidobacteria, which is why I recommend a probiotic supplement that contains both Lacto and Bifido. Recently, many new probiotic products have appeared on store shelves and in supplements, foods, beverages—even chewing gum. With all the variety, it can be difficult to determine which products are of high quality.

> **The participants of the Skinny Gut Diet began by taking 50 billion cultures of probiotics daily and increased the dosage to 100 billion daily after six weeks. Their digestion and gut balance improved, and their weight came off.**

What to look for in a probiotic:

- High culture count: This number refers to the total amount of bacteria per capsule. Look for a probiotics supplement with at least 30 billion cultures.
- Number of strains: Your supplement should include at least ten different strains of bacteria scientifically studied to benefit optimal health. Look for high amounts of *Bifidobacterium* to support the large intestine (colon) and *Lactobacillus* to support the small intestine and urogenital tract. Remember—look for the Ls and the Bs.
- Targeted- and delayed-release capsules: These capsules protect the probiotics from harsh stomach acid and deliver them directly to the intestines, where they are needed and utilized by the body.
- Potency guarantee: The potency, or amount of live cultures, should be guaranteed though time of expiration under recom-

mended storage conditions. Many products guarantee potency only through time of manufacture, which means that you don't know how much you are really getting by the time you take it.

- See the Resources, page 255, for my product recommendations.

Dosage:

Take a high-potency, multistrain probiotic daily.

What to Look for in a Probiotic Supplement:

	Amount per Serving
Probiotic Blend	
Bifidobacterium lactis	
Bifidobacterium breve	
Bifidobacterium longum	
Lactobacillus acidophilus	
Lactobacillus casei	
Lactobacillus plantarum	
Lactobacillus paracasei	
Lactobacillus salivarius	
Lactobacillus rhamnosus	
Lactobacillus bulgaricus	
Total Bifido/Lacto Cultures	**50 billion**

E is for Enzymes

Enzymes play an essential role in every function of the human body. In the digestive system, enzymes break apart the bonds that hold nutrients together so the body can use those nutrients for energy. This is what we think of as digestion.

If your food isn't broken down, the nutrients won't be absorbed and your immune system may respond to the unrecognizable food particles as if they were foreign enemies, mounting a fight against them that produces silent inflammation and unpleasant symptoms of gas, bloating, and other digestive upsets. Reducing the inflammation in the gut is an important way to maintain gut bacterial balance.

"When I take enzymes, my midriff doesn't feel bloated and puffy like before." —Cynthia

Although enzymes are present in raw, whole foods, most of us don't get enough enzymes through diet alone. The cooking and processing of foods removes necessary enzymes, and improper chewing or eating habits can impact your body's ability to digest your meal. Several locations in the digestive system secrete enzymes, but only when your digestive system is operating efficiently. And production of enzymes decreases with age. Also, there are some enzymes that the body doesn't create, which is why many people have difficulty digesting beans, legumes, and nuts. Taking a digestive enzyme with every meal (and snacks if you want to get extra digestive benefit) will help ensure that your body is breaking your food down into usable nutrients and you have a healthy gut.

What to look for in a digestive enzyme supplement:

- High-potency plant-based enzyme formula
- Targeted-delivery capsules (see above)
- High Enzyme Activity Value (EAV), a measure of enzyme potency that determines how well the enzymes break down each food group
- Varied enzyme blend for full-spectrum digestion. Look for an array of plant-based enzymes in addition to protease, lipase, and amylase.
- Look for the IZYME seal to ensure you are getting a high-potency, purified digestive enzyme supplement.
- See Resources, page 255, for my product recommendations.

Dosage:
Take high-potency digestive enzymes with each meal.

What to Look for in a Digestive Enzyme Supplement:

	Amount per Serving
Plant-based Enzyme Blend	
Protein Enzyme Activity Value	2,300,000 PU
Papain, Bromelain, Protease SP, Protease PC, Peptidase, Protease DP, Protease AP, Actinidin	
Carbohydrate Enzyme Activity Value	40,000 DP
Amylase Blend, Lactase, Invertase, Alpha Galactosidase, Maltase, Glucoamylase, Phytase	
Fat Enzyme Activity Value	4,300 FIP
Lipase Blend	
Fiber Enzyme Activity Value	4,100 CU
Cellulase Blend, Hemicellulase, Xylanase, Beta Glucanase, Pectinase	

Meal-Replacement Shake

In addition to those in the H.O.P.E. Formula, a supplement that will be helpful for you while on the Skinny Gut Diet is a meal-replacement shake. These shakes can be used to replace meals or be snacks. It's an easy way to get your protein, fiber, and nutrients when you're on the go. Look for a meal-replacement shake that contains 20 grams of protein and 10 grams of fiber. In addition, look for a plant-based shake with a variety of plant proteins, including pea protein, along with a plant fiber complex of acacia fiber, flax or chia seeds, and hemp. Finally, make sure your meal-replacement shake includes digestive enzymes and probiotics.

What to look for in a meal-replacement shake:

- 20 grams of protein
- 10 grams of fiber
- Gluten-free, no added sugar
- Organic, grain-free, plant-based protein and fiber blend featuring pea, hemp, sacha inchi, acacia, and flax
- Added *Bifidobacterium* and *Lactobacillus* probiotics
- Added digestive enzymes

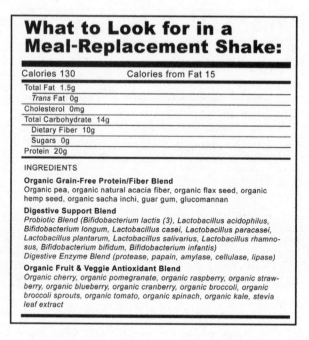

What to Look for in a Meal-Replacement Shake:

Calories 130	Calories from Fat 15

Total Fat 1.5g
   Trans Fat 0g
Cholesterol 0mg
Total Carbohydrate 14g
   Dietary Fiber 10g
   Sugars 0g
Protein 20g

INGREDIENTS

Organic Grain-Free Protein/Fiber Blend
Organic pea, organic natural acacia fiber, organic flax seed, organic hemp seed, organic sacha inchi, guar gum, glucomannan

Digestive Support Blend
Probiotic Blend (Bifidobacterium lactis (3), Lactobacillus acidophilus, Bifidobacterium longum, Lactobacillus casei, Lactobacillus paracasei, Lactobacillus plantarum, Lactobacillus salivarius, Lactobacillus rhamnosus, Bifidobacterium bifidum, Bifidobacterium infantis)
Digestive Enzyme Blend (protease, papain, amylase, cellulase, lipase)

Organic Fruit & Veggie Antioxidant Blend
Organic cherry, organic pomegranate, organic raspberry, organic strawberry, organic blueberry, organic cranberry, organic broccoli, organic broccoli sprouts, organic tomato, organic spinach, organic kale, stevia leaf extract

CHAPTER 11 SUMMARY

H.O.P.E. Formula

➤ **H is for High Fiber:** Take a fiber supplement in the morning and at night along with a glass of water. Fiber can also be taken before meals to reduce hunger.

➤ **O is for Omega-3:** Take at least 2,000 mg of total omega-3 daily. (Be sure that you are taking 2,000 mg of omega-3 and not just 2,000 mg of fish oil.)

➤ **P is for Probiotics:** Take a high-potency, multistrain probiotic daily.

➤ **E is for Enzymes:** Take digestive enzymes with each meal.

Meal-Replacement Shake

➤ Enjoy a meal-replacement shake as a meal or snack on a regular basis.

Chapter 12

THE STAY LEAN PHASE

Congratulations! You have reached your ideal weight. Now it's time to refine your eating habits so that you can maintain your skinny gut for life. As I have said throughout this book, the Skinny Gut Diet is a *new way of eating*. It's not just a diet. It teaches you how to view food differently—and to choose food differently. You'll get that skinny gut you've always wanted and—most important—you'll keep it for good.

Find the Right Sugar Balance for a Lifetime of Skinny

Here's the formula: Once you reach your desired weight, you can add 2 teaspoons of sugar to your daily total so that your target is between 10 and 12 teaspoons of sugar daily from the foods you eat. You eat that way for a month. If you do not gain back any weight or do not experience any digestive symptoms—or if you continue to lose weight—you increase by 2 more teaspoons your intake of sugar from all the foods you eat. You continue using the Teaspoon Tracker calculation just as you have been doing, and you eat that way for another month. You add 2 teaspoons of sugar to your total each month, until you begin to gain weight or experience symptoms. At that point, you will know you need to decrease your daily teaspoons of sugar by 2 in order to maintain your optimal weight for life.

Some people will be able to add more sugar to their total than others. That's because people vary. You may be able to eat food that adds up to 14 to 16 teaspoons daily, while your best friend may have to keep it to between 10 and 12. It all depends on how your body uses insulin. The STAY LEAN PHASE is designed to help you find your perfect sugar intake so that your gut stays balanced and you stay skinny.

RULE 1

EAT MORE FAT (*HEALTHY* FAT) TO REDUCE SILENT INFLAMMATION

In the STAY LEAN PHASE, Rule 1 remains exactly the same. You continue to eat healthy fats and minimize unhealthy fats, just as you did during the GET LEAN PHASE. By now you will have developed the habit of cooking and baking with coconut and olive oils, and using extra-virgin olive oil or flaxseed oil for salads, sauces, and dips. You will eat plenty of foods naturally high in healthy fats, and you will feel comfortable eating saturated fats in moderation.

RULE 2

EAT LIVING FOODS EVERY DAY TO BALANCE YOUR GUT

In the STAY LEAN PHASE, you continue to eat living foods every day, but you will be able to add certain foods like beans, grains, and additional fruits in small amounts. Because your total teaspoons of sugar (including hidden sugar) from all the foods you eat will increase in increments of 2 teaspoons at a time, you will add only small amounts of these foods while remaining within your sugar goal.

The following list will help you determine what foods you can add and how much you can add.

FOODS YOU CAN ADD	tsp sugar
Beans	
1 cup cooked black bean pasta	1.2
1 cup cooked mung bean pasta	1.5
½ cup cooked black beans	2.6
½ cup cooked kidney beans	2.9
½ cup cooked navy beans	2.9
½ cup cooked pinto beans	3.0
½ cup cooked garbanzo beans	3.3
Vegetables	
Yam, ½ cup	3.6

FOODS YOU CAN ADD	tsp sugar
Grains	
½ cup cooked black rice	1.5
½ cup cooked oats (gluten free)	2.7
½ cup cooked quinoa	3.4
½ cup cooked couscous	3.4
½ cup cooked millet	3.9
Fruits	
Pomegranate, ½ cup	2.6
Honeydew melon, 1 cup diced	2.8
Tangerine, 1 large	2.8
Orange, 1 large	3.6

Although you avoided grains in the GET LEAN PHASE, you may find that you can tolerate small amounts of grains in the STAY LEAN PHASE, if—and this is a big *if*—you do not begin to gain weight and you do not experience any health symptoms. Not only do grains contribute to an ever-widening waistline but certain grains—wheat and corn, in particular—can lead to or worsen many health conditions. If bread, pasta, rice, cereal, cakes, muffins, and pastries are your comfort foods, you crave them for a reason: the fat-promoting bacteria thrive on them. On top of that, you may be sensitive to wheat or corn, which are substances found in virtually all processed foods. If you find that you can tolerate grains without a return of symptoms or a surge in your weight, then limit your intake to *no more than ½ cup daily*. (Remember that 1 cup of cooked brown rice is a whopping 8.2 teaspoons of sugar, so ½ cup is 4.1 teaspoons. If you eat ½ cup of cooked quinoa, you'll add 3.4 teaspoons of sugar to your daily total, so you may be better off limiting your grains to ¼ cup.) But don't worry, I have good news. In Chapter 13, you will find some delicious recipes that will satisfy your sweet tooth. You won't even miss the sugar-laden versions once you've tried these treats. And if you miss your pasta, I've got more good news. See Resources, page 254, for my recommendations on a delicious, low-carb pasta you will enjoy.

In the GET LEAN PHASE, you did not eat wheat or gluten, so as to avoid any roadblocks on the journey toward achieving excellent digestive health. In the STAY LEAN PHASE, you are best served by continuing to avoid gluten, with the exception of the occasional dinner out, catered event, or accidental encounter. Wheat and gluten are troublesome when it comes to keeping off weight. A little gluten here or there won't hurt (unless you have celiac disease or a gluten sensitivity, of course), but it can interfere with your progress toward weight loss. If you are in a pinch, and it's a matter of eating a dinner that has a tiny amount of gluten in the sauce thickener, eat the dinner.

RULE 3

EAT PROTEIN AT EVERY MEAL AND SNACK TO ELIMINATE CRAVINGS

As you did during the GET LEAN PHASE, you continue to eat protein throughout the day to control any cravings. Because some protein foods will be included in your total teaspoons of sugar, you will be able to eat more of these foods while staying within your daily limit. By now you are accustomed to eating protein at every meal and snack, so you will find the STAY LEAN PHASE an easy transition. And remember: you are creating a new way of eating. The Skinny Gut Diet is a lifestyle guide, not a short-term weight-loss trick. It's about establishing new habits that you will keep for life. It's about eating healthy and feeling your best.

STAY LEAN PHASE Summary

During the STAY LEAN PHASE you eat foods that add up to at least 10 to 12 teaspoons of sugar daily while following the three simple rules:

Rule 1: Eat more fat (healthy fat) to reduce silent inflammation.
Rule 2: Eat living foods every day to balance your gut.

Rule 3: Eat protein at every meal and snack to eliminate cravings.

You will add 2 teaspoons of sugar to your total each month until you start to gain weight or experience digestive symptoms. You will then back off 2 teaspoons of sugar and keep this as your daily target. Everybody is different. This phase is personalized for your body and gut type.

To give you an idea of what eating during the STAY LEAN PHASE looks like, consider this sample day.

MEAL	INGREDIENTS	tsp sugar
Breakfast		1.4
Meal-Replacement Shake (page 146)	Meal-Replacement Shake + 1 cup unsweetened almond milk	
Snack		0
Turkey cheese roll-up	2 ounce turkey slice + 1 ounce Cheddar cheese + romaine leaf	
Lunch		4
Panera lunch	You Pick Two: Turkey Chili and Classic Salad	
Snack		0.6
Almonds and pumpkin seeds	14 almonds + ¼ cup raw pumpkin seeds	
Dinner		4.8
Thyme-Stuffed Steak on Cress (page 203) with quinoa salad	Thyme-Stuffed Steak on Cress + ¼ cup cooked quinoa + ½ avocado + 8 cherry tomatoes + 2 cups spring mix + ¼ cup sauerkraut	
Snack		1.4
Whipped Cream Sundae (page 141)	¼ cup whipped cream + ¼ cup blueberries + ⅛ cup walnuts	
TOTAL	**9 servings**	**12.2**

I would love to hear your story. If you have found success with the Skinny Gut Diet, as I know you will, please share your experience with me. Visit skinnygutdiet.com and sign up to access the site, receive updates, and submit your Skinny Gut story.

CHAPTER 12 SUMMARY

Once you reach your desired weight, you increase your daily consumption of sugar in increments of 2 teaspoons. If you do not gain any weight or do not experience any digestive symptoms, or if you continue to lose weight, you continue to increase your intake of sugar by 2 teaspoons. You use the Teaspoon Tracker calculation, and eat that way for another month. You continue adding 2 teaspoons of sugar to your total each month until you begin to gain weight or experience symptoms.

You follow the same three simple rules of the diet:

Rule 1: Eat more fat (healthy fat) to reduce silent inflammation.
➤ Rule 1 remains exactly the same. You continue to eat healthy fats and minimize unhealthy fats.

Rule 2: Eat living foods every day to balance your gut.
➤ You continue to eat living foods every day, but you are able to add certain foods like beans, grains, and fruits in small amounts.

Rule 3: Eat protein at every meal and snack to eliminate cravings.
➤ You continue to eat protein throughout the day to control cravings.

Chapter 13

FOOD AND RECIPES TO GET YOU STARTED

Now that you know the three simple rules of the Skinny Gut Diet, here is everything you need to put what you have learned into action. This chapter includes a two-week meal plan to give you an idea of how to eat throughout the week. It will also help guide your own planning process beyond that week. You can either follow the meal plans to a tee, or improvise with your own modifications that fit your personal goal for maximum teaspoons of sugar.

The recipes are designed to be used in either phase of the diet. Each recipe indicates the total teaspoons of sugar per serving, so that you can easily track your sugar intake. I've already done the calculation for you! In Chapter 14, you will find more tools to help you implement the diet successfully (and what to do in alternative situations, such as eating out or attending a dinner party).

SKINNY GUT DIET TWO-WEEK MEAL PLANNER: WEEK I

	Breakfast	Snack	Lunch
Sunday	Mini Spinach Omelets (page 181) + ½ cup strawberries	2 celery ribs with almond butter	Brenda's Egg Salad (page 187) over 1 cup romaine lettuce
Tsp sugar	1.5	1	1.2
Monday	2 eggs, any style, 2 slices of turkey bacon, side of blueberries	Plain Greek yogurt	Brenda's Chicken Salad (page 187) with Natural Creamy Dressing (page 189) over 1 cup salad greens
Tsp sugar	2.4	1.7	1.3
Tuesday	Plain Greek yogurt with blackberries	Handful of nuts	Chicken Lime Cobb Salad (page 185)
Tsp sugar	1.8	0.4	2
Wednesday	Meal-Replacement Shake (page 146) + ½ cup strawberries	Turkey jerky, 3 pieces	Unstuffed Cabbage (page 215) leftovers
Tsp sugar	1.5	0.4	3.4
Thursday	Veggie scramble (2 eggs plus non-starchy veggies)	Turkey-Guac Roll-Ups (page 141)	Chicken tenders + 1 cup steamed broccoli + 1 ounce Cheddar cheese + ⅛ cup sunflower seeds
Tsp sugar	1.4	0.4	0.8
Friday	2 eggs, any style, 2 slices of turkey bacon, side of blueberries	Baby carrots and hummus, ½ cup of each	Chicken sausage meatballs + spinach salad
Tsp sugar	2.4	2	0.7
Saturday	Veggie Egg Patties (page 185) + ½ cup strawberries	Shelled edamame, ½ cup	Meal-Replacement Shake (page 146) + ½ cup strawberries
Tsp sugar	1.1	0.8	1.5

Snack	Anytime	Dinner	Snack	TOTAL
Cottage cheese, 4 ounces + ¼ cup pineapple	½ cup fermented vegetables, any kind	Chicken Milanese (page 208)	Berries-n-Cream (page 223)	**Sunday**
1.8	0.5	1.2	2.1	**9.3**
Shelled edamame, ½ cup	½ cup fermented vegetables, any kind	Persian Kebabs (page 204)	Cacao, Avocado, and Chia Mousse (page 225)	**Monday**
0.8	0.5	0.8	0.6	**8.1**
Roll-ups (3): slice of deli meat + slice of cheese + lettuce leaf	½ cup fermented vegetables, any kind	Unstuffed Cabbage (page 215)	Coco-Nut Pudding (page 225)	**Tuesday**
0	0.5	3.4	0.6	**8.7**
Turkey slices, 2 ounces with cheese	½ caup fermented vegetables, any kind	Meat and Veggie Bolognese (page 205)	Joy's Lemon Bliss (page 224)	**Wednesday**
0.4	0.5	2.2	0.2	**8.6**
Turkey-Hummus Roll-Ups (page 141)	½ cup plain kefir	Lemongrass Chicken (page 207)	Berries-n-Cream (page 223)	**Thursday**
2	1.2	1.6	2.1	**8.7**
Plain Greek yogurt	½ cup plain kefir	Sicilian Citrus Pork (page 206)	Nut Butter Chocolate Cups (page 224)	**Friday**
1.7	1.2	0.6	0.2	**8.8**
Turkey-Hummus Roll-Ups (page 141)	½ cup fermented vegetables, any kind	Ligurian Chicken (page 214)	Nut Butter Chocolate Cups (page 224)	**Saturday**
1.2	0.5	3.6	0.2	**8.9**

SKINNY GUT DIET TWO-WEEK MEAL PLANNER: WEEK 2

	Breakfast	Snack	Lunch
Sunday	Veggie scramble (2 eggs plus nonstarchy veggies) + ½ cup strawberries	Plain Greek yogurt	Brenda's Chicken Salad (page 187) over 1 cup romaine, ½ cup red pepper
Tsp Sugar	1.9	1.7	1.7
Monday	Plain Greek yogurt with blackberries	Roll-ups (3): slice of deli meat + slice of cheese + lettuce leaf	Tuna Salad (page 188) + Natural Creamy Dressing (page 189)
Tsp Sugar	1.9	0	1.1
Tuesday	Meal-Replacement Shake (page 146) + ½ cup strawberries	Baby carrots and hummus, ½ cup of each	Smoked Salmon Salad (page 188) over 1 cup mixed greens
Tsp Sugar	1.5	2	0.2
Wednesday	Pam's Egg Frittatas (page 182) + ½ cup black berries	Cucumber canoes (page 140)	Slow Cooker Chicken Parmigiana (page 150) leftovers
Tsp Sugar	1.8	1.1	1.3
Thursday	Spinach and Goat Cheese Omelet (page 184)	4 oz cottage cheese + ½ cup blackberries	Chicken in a Lettuce Bowl (page 210)
Tsp Sugar	1.2	1.3	1
Friday	Salmon Frittata (page 183)	Turkey jerky, 3 pieces	Meal-Replacement Shake (page 146) + ½ cup strawberries
Tsp Sugar	2	0.4	1.5
Saturday	Veggie scramble (2 eggs plus non-starchy veggies) + ½ cup strawberries	Shelled edamame, ½ cup	Slow Cooker Chicken Cacciatore (page 149) leftovers
Tsp Sugar	1.9	0.8	1.5

Snack	Anytime	Dinner	Snack	TOTAL
2 celery ribs with almond butter	½ cup fermented vegetables, any kind	Salmon with ½ cup broccoli + ½ cup cauliflower	Berries-n-Cream (page 223)	**Sunday**
0.2	0.5	0.8	2.1	**8.9**
½ Granny Smith apple + 1 tablespoon nut butter	½ cup plain kefir	Beef Bruschetta (page 192)	Strawberry Kefir Ice Cream (page 226)	**Monday**
2	1.2	1.4	0.7	**8.3**
Handful of nuts	½ cup plain kefir	Slow Cooker Chicken Parmigiana (page 150)	Berries-n-Cream (page 223)	**Tuesday**
0.4	1.2	1.3	2.1	**8.7**
Roast Beef and Asparagus Roll-Up (page 140)	½ cup fermented vegetables, any kind	Turkey Burgers (page 215) over mixed greens + ½ cup red bell peppers + handful of nuts	Cacao, Avocado, and Chia Mousse (page 225)	**Wednesday**
0.6	0.5	2.7	0.6	**8.6**
Plain Greek yogurt	½ cup fermented vegetables, any kind	Baked Fish (page 200) + 1 cup summer squash	Whipped Cream Sundae (page 141)	**Thursday**
1.7	0.5	2	1.4	**9.1**
Roll-ups (3): slice of deli meat + slice of cheese + lettuce leaf	½ cup fermented vegetables, any kind	Slow Cooker Chicken Cacciatore (page 149)	Coco-Nut Pudding (page 225)	**Friday**
0	0.5	3	0.6	**8**
2 celery ribs with Roasted Red Pepper Hummus (page 142)	½ cup plain kefir	Chicken Asparagus Stir-Fry (page 213)	Nut Butter Chocolate Cups (page 224)	**Saturday**
1.5	1.2	1.4	0.2	**8.5**

BREAKFASTS

NUTMEAL

2.3 teaspoons sugar
15 minutes to prepare and cook
Serves 3

¼ cup raw cashews
¼ cup walnuts
¼ cup pecans
1 teaspoon ground cinnamon
¼ teaspoon ground ginger
3 tablespoons flax seeds
1 large egg
½ cup unsweetened almond or coconut milk
1 tablespoon almond butter
Butter or nondairy spread
Fresh blackberries

1. Combine the nuts, spices, and flax seeds in a food processor or blender. Blend until the mixture has a coarse-grain texture.

2. Whisk the egg and almond milk. Mix the ground nuts and almond butter into the egg and milk mixture

3. Heat the mixture in a saucepan over medium heat until it's the desired consistency, 3 to 4 minutes. Stir frequently. Serve topped with 1 teaspoon butter or nondairy spread and blackberries.

TURKEY SAUSAGE PATTIES

0.1 teaspoon sugar
20 minutes to prepare and cook, 1 hour to chill
Serves 3

1 pound ground turkey
1 teaspoon dried sage

½ teaspoon fennel seeds
2 garlic cloves
½ teaspoon salt
Dash of freshly ground black pepper
Dash of cayenne
Dash of ground allspice

1. Combine all the ingredients in a medium bowl. Shape into twelve 3-inch patties and refrigerate for at least 1 hour.
2. Cook the patties for 4 to 6 minutes on each side, until cooked through.

MINI SPINACH OMELETS

0.7 teaspoon sugar
30 minutes to prepare and cook
Serves 6

2 teaspoons coconut oil
½ cup chopped onion
½ cup sliced button mushrooms
1 cup chopped baby spinach
4 large eggs
2 tablespoons almond milk
Salt and freshly ground black pepper

1. Preheat the oven to 350°F. Coat a mini muffin pan with a little coconut oil.
2. Heat the oil in a sauté pan on medium heat. Sauté the onion and mushrooms until soft, about 5 minutes. Add the spinach and cook until just wilted, about 1 minute more. Remove the pan from the heat and let cool.
3. Whisk the eggs and almond milk in a medium bowl. Add the spinach mixture, then pour into the cups of the muffin pan, filling the cups about halfway.
4. Bake for 15 to 20 minutes, or until set.

PAM'S EGG FRITTATAS

0.5 teaspoon sugar
20 minutes to prepare and cook
Serves 12

2 teaspoons coconut oil
½ orange bell pepper, chopped
½ yellow bell pepper, chopped
1 shallot, chopped
1 tablespoon Italian seasoning
12 large eggs
½ cup milk
½ cup shredded Cheddar cheese
½ cup grated Parmesan cheese
Salt and freshly ground black pepper

1. Preheat the oven to 350°F. Heat the oil in a medium sauté pan. Add the bell peppers and shallot and sauté until tender but not brown. Add the seasoning. Let cool.

2. Beat the eggs and milk in a bowl until fluffy, 2 to 3 minutes. Stir in the pepper mixture, cheeses, and salt and pepper.

3. Lightly coat a 12-muffin pan with coconut oil.

4. Pour the egg mixture into the muffin pan, filling the cups about three-quarters full. Place in the oven and bake for 20 to 30 minutes, until lightly golden brown on top.

SALMON FRITTATA

2.0 teaspoons sugar
30 minutes to prepare and cook
Serves 2

1 teaspoon coconut oil
¼ cup diced sweet onion
¼ cup frozen or fresh steamed corn kernels
One 4-ounce can salmon, drained
1 ripe tomato, diced
¼ cup chopped red bell pepper
2 large eggs, lightly beaten
4 cups trimmed fresh spinach
¼ cup sliced avocado
¼ cup of your favorite salsa
1 tablespoon chopped fresh mint or basil leaves
Pinch of salt
Freshly ground black pepper
3 tablespoons grated Cheddar cheese (optional)

1. Preheat the broiler. In a large ovenproof skillet, heat the coconut oil over medium heat. Cook the onion until softened, about 3 minutes. Add the corn, salmon, tomato, and bell pepper. Gently stir to combine, and continue to cook for about 4 minutes more.

2. Pour the eggs over the mixture. Cook on medium heat for about 4 minutes more.

3. Place the skillet in the broiler and broil for 1 to 2 minutes, until the eggs are light golden brown on top. Watch carefully.

4. Cut the frittata into wedges and serve on a bed of spinach topped with fanned avocado slices and salsa. Sprinkle with the fresh herbs, salt, and pepper. Top with cheese, if desired.

SPINACH AND GOAT CHEESE OMELET

1.2 teaspoons sugar
30 minutes to prepare and cook
Serves 1

2 large eggs, lightly beaten
2 teaspoons coconut oil
2 cups firmly packed baby spinach
¼ cup diced sweet onion
½ cup frozen artichokes, thawed and roughly chopped
¼ cup goat cheese
Salt and freshly ground black pepper

1. Lightly beat the eggs in a small bowl. Heat 1 teaspoon of the coconut oil in a 9-inch sauté pan set over medium-high heat. Add the spinach and stir, cooking for 1 to 2 minutes, only until slightly wilted. Remove from the pan and place in a bowl.

2. Heat the remaining 1 teaspoon coconut oil in the skillet over medium heat. Add the onion and artichokes, and sauté for 2 minutes until slightly tender.

3. Stir in the eggs, let cook 1 minute to set, and gently lift the edges to allow the remaining liquid egg slide underneath. Cook for 3 to 4 minutes more, until the omelet is firm. Flip the omelet and immediately spread all but 1 teaspoon of the goat cheese on top. Cover with the wilted spinach and continue to cook on low heat for 2 minutes.

4. Fold the omelet in half and remove from the pan, sliding it onto a plate. Serve with the remaining goat cheese. Season with salt and pepper to taste.

VEGGIE EGG PATTIES

0.6 teaspoon sugar
30 minutes to prepare and cook
Serves 3

1 large egg
1 zucchini, grated
1 red bell pepper, seeded and grated
½ onion, chopped
Salt and freshly ground black pepper
3 tablespoons coconut oil

1. In a mixing bowl, whisk the egg lightly and add the zucchini, bell pepper, and onion. Add salt and pepper to taste.

2. Heat the coconut oil in a sauté pan over medium heat. Form three patties of the veggie-egg mixture and place in the pan. Sauté for about 3 minutes on each side, until lightly browned.

SALADS

CHICKEN LIME COBB SALAD

2 teaspoons sugar
15 minutes to prepare
Serves 2

Dressing
2 teaspoons extra-virgin olive oil
¼ cup buttermilk
2 teaspoons minced jarred pickled jalapeño pepper
Juice of 1 lime
2 teaspoons Dijon-style mustard

Salad

8 ounces cooked chicken breast, chopped

½ red bell pepper, chopped

½ green bell pepper, chopped

¼ red onion, chopped

1 ripe tomato, chopped

½ avocado, scooped out and chopped

¼ cup reduced-fat blue cheese crumbles

1 hard-boiled egg, chopped

2 cups mixed salad greens

1. For the dressing: In a small bowl, whisk together all the ingredients.

2. For the salad: In a large bowl, combine all the salad ingredients. Drizzle on the dressing and serve.

CRAB AND WHITE BEAN SALAD

1.8 teaspoons sugar

30 minutes to prepare and chill

Serves 4

⅓ cup chopped yellow pepper

¼ cup chopped red onion

¼ cup chopped celery

1 tablespoon white wine vinegar

½ tablespoon fresh lime juice

½ tablespoon extra-virgin olive oil

Dash of hot sauce

One 6-ounce can lump crab meat, drained

1 cup cooked cannellini beans, drained and rinsed

3 cups chopped salad greens

Combine all the ingredients except the greens in a large bowl; toss gently. Cover and chill for 30 minutes. Serve over the greens.

BRENDA'S EGG SALAD

0.2 teaspoon sugar
30 minutes to prepare and chill
Serves 1

2 hard-boiled eggs
½ teaspoon prepared mustard
½ tablespoon mayonnaise
½ tablespoon pickle relish
2 tablespoons chopped celery
1 teaspoon celery seeds
Freshly ground black pepper

Place the eggs in a small bowl and mash with a fork. Add the remaining ingredients and mix well. Chill for 20 minutes and enjoy alone, inside a lettuce leaf wrap, or with salad.

BRENDA'S CHICKEN SALAD

0.3 teaspoon sugar
1 hour 30 minutes to prepare, cook, and chill
Serves 8

One 3-pound chicken, rinsed
1 onion, chopped
1 tablespoon minced garlic
6 tablespoons mayonnaise
2 ribs celery, chopped
¼ cup pecans or walnuts
½ Granny Smith apple
Salt and freshly ground black pepper

1. Place the chicken and onion in a stockpot and cover with water. Bring to a boil, turn the heat down, and simmer on medium heat for about 1 hour or until the meat is falling off the bones. Let cool.

2. Remove the meat from the bones and shred. Mix the shredded chicken with the other ingredients and chill for 20 minutes.

3. Serve plain, inside a lettuce leaf wrap, or with salad greens.

TUNA SALAD

0.4 teaspoon sugar
25 minutes to prepare and chill
Serves 1

One 6-ounce can light tuna in water, drained
1 tablespoon mayonnaise
½ tablespoon pickle relish
2 slices Granny Smith apple, chopped
½ teaspoon celery seeds
Freshly ground black pepper

Mix all the ingredients in a medium bowl and chill for 20 minutes. Serve plain, inside a lettuce leaf wrap, or with salad greens.

SMOKED SALMON SALAD

0 teaspoon sugar
25 minutes to prepare and chill
Serves 1

One 4-ounce fillet of smoked salmon
1 rib celery
2 tablespoons mayonnaise
1 tablespoon drained capers
Freshly ground black pepper

Flake the salmon into a medium bowl. Add the remaining ingredients and mix well. Chill for 20 minutes. Serve plain, inside a lettuce leaf wrap, or with salad greens.

JICAMA BEET SALAD

1.3 teaspoons sugar

15 minutes to prepare

Serves 4

    ½ large jicama, peeled and julienned

    1 cooked red beet, peeled and julienned

    1 cooked golden beet, peeled and julienned

    1 tablespoon lime juice

    ½ teaspoon ground ginger

    Salt

    Mint leaves, for garnish

Place all the ingredients in a bowl and stir. Garnish with the mint, if desired, and serve as a side dish.

Dressings

NATURAL CREAMY DRESSING

0.7 teaspoon sugar

5 minutes to prepare

Makes 8 servings

    1 cup plain Greek yogurt

    1 avocado, pulp scooped out

    ½ lemon

    ¼ teaspoon minced garlic

    1 tablespoon chopped fresh parsley

    Salt and freshly ground black pepper

    Pinch of red pepper flakes (optional)

Add all the ingredients to a blender or food processor and spin until smooth.

NATURAL RANCH DRESSING

0.8 teaspoon sugar
5 minutes to prepare
Makes 1 serving

1 tablespoon plain Greek yogurt
1 tablespoon balsamic or rice vinegar
1 tablespoon stone-ground mustard
¼ teaspoon lo han (monk fruit) sweetener (see Resources, page 256)

Combine all the ingredients in a small bowl and mix with a fork.

NATURAL MUSTARD VINAIGRETTE DRESSING

0 teaspoon sugar
5 minutes to prepare
Makes 1 serving

2 tablespoons extra-virgin olive oil
1 tablespoon spicy mustard
½ teaspoon red wine vinegar
¼ teaspoon freshly ground black pepper

Place all the ingredients in a small bowl and mix with a fork.

STARTERS

GARLIC-N-LEMON SHRIMP

1.4 teaspoons sugar
30 minutes to prepare and cook
Serves 2

12 garlic cloves
1 tablespoon coconut oil

1 pound large shrimp (21–25 count), peeled and deveined

½ teaspoon smoked paprika

¼ teaspoon red pepper flakes

Juice of 1 lemon

1 tablespoon chopped fresh parsley

1. Preheat the oven to 375°F. Combine the whole garlic and oil in a small ovenproof skillet and bake, uncovered, for 15 to 20 minutes, stirring occasionally, until golden brown.

2. Remove the garlic from the oil and set aside. Transfer the oil in the skillet to a large sauté pan and heat over medium-high heat. Add the shrimp, paprika, and red pepper flakes and sauté the shrimp for about 3 minutes per side, until they turn pink. Add the baked garlic and sauté for 1 minute.

3. Toss the shrimp with lemon juice and parsley, and serve.

SEARED SESAME TUNA

1 teaspoon sugar

45 minutes to prepare and cook

Serves 4

Slaw (0.8 teaspoon sugar)

1 tablespoon dark sesame oil

1 tablespoon tamari

1 tablespoon mirin

1 tablespoon rice wine vinegar (sugar-free)

2 teaspoons minced fresh ginger

1 garlic clove, minced

½ teaspoon red pepper flakes

3 cups thinly sliced Napa cabbage

1 cup thinly sliced bok choy

½ red bell pepper, thinly sliced

1 carrot, thinly sliced

3 scallions, green and white parts thinly sliced

Tuna (0.2 teaspoon sugar)

   1 tablespoon white sesame seeds

   ½ tablespoon black sesame seeds

   ¼ teaspoon wasabi powder

   1 pound tuna steak, about 2 inches thick

   1 teaspoon coconut oil

   1 tablespoon minced fresh cilantro

1. For the slaw: In a small bowl, whisk together the sesame oil, tamari, mirin, vinegar, ginger, garlic, and red pepper flakes.

2. In a large bowl, combine the cabbage, bok choy, red pepper slices, carrot, and scallions. Add the dressing and mix well. Set aside for at least 20 minutes.

3. For the tuna: In a shallow bowl, combine the sesame seeds and wasabi. Coat the tuna steaks in the sesame seed mixture, making sure both sides are covered.

4. Heat the coconut oil in a large skillet over medium-high heat. Sear the tuna in the pan for 2 to 3 minutes per side, until both sides are well browned but the tuna is still very rare in the center.

5. Garnish the tuna with the cilantro and serve with the slaw.

BEEF BRUSCHETTA

1.4 teaspoons sugar
30 minutes to prepare and cook
Serves 2

   3 teaspoons coconut oil

   ½ cup halved artichoke hearts (packed in water)

   ¼ red onion, minced

   1 ripe tomato, diced

   3 fresh basil leaves, minced

   1 garlic clove, minced

   1 tablespoon balsamic vinegar

8 ounces lean boneless beef (top round or sirloin), cut into ½-inch
   slices
½ teaspoon cracked black peppercorns
¼ teaspoon Italian seasoning

1. Coat a grill pan or cast-iron skillet with 2 teaspoons of the
coconut oil and heat over medium-high heat. Lightly brown the artichoke hearts on each side, 2 to 3 minutes. Remove from the heat,
cool, then cut into smaller pieces.

2. In a small bowl, combine the artichoke hearts, onion, tomato,
remaining 1 teaspoon coconut oil, basil, garlic, and vinegar.

3. Season the beef with the cracked peppercorns and Italian seasoning, patting to coat the sides of each slice. In the same grill pan or
cast-iron skillet, sear the beef slices over medium-high heat for about
2 minutes per side, until nicely browned. Transfer to a plate and top
with the artichoke mixture.

ATHENIAN MEATBALLS

0.6 teaspoon sugar
55 minutes to prepare and cook
Serves 6

1 white onion, quartered
¼ cup fresh dill sprigs
¼ cup fresh mint leaves
2 garlic cloves
½ cup grated zucchini
1 pound ground lamb
1 large egg, beaten
¼ cup crumbled feta cheese
¼ teaspoon freshly ground black pepper
2 tablespoons water or nonfat milk

1. Preheat the oven to 375°F. Place the onion, dill, mint, and garlic in a food processor and pulse 8 to 12 times, until chopped and well mixed. Add the zucchini and pulse 2 or 3 times more to combine. Transfer the mixture to a large bowl.

2. Add the lamb, egg, cheese, and pepper and mix with your hands until well combined. Wet your hands with water or milk and form the mixture into balls slightly larger than a golf ball.

3. Heat a large skillet over medium-high heat. Brown the meatballs for 5 minutes all around, then place on an ovenproof dish or pan. Place in the oven on the center rack and bake for about 30 minutes.

GRILLED CHICKEN KEBABS

0.6 teaspoon sugar
25 minutes to prepare and cook, 2 hours to marinate
Serves 4

3 boneless, skinless chicken breast halves, cut into large cubes
12 cherry tomatoes
12 medium button mushrooms, halved
1 garlic clove, minced
Zest of ½ lemon
1 tablespoon fresh lemon juice
1 tablespoon olive oil
½ tablespoon fresh oregano leaves, chopped

1. Soak four wooden skewers in water for 30 minutes to prevent burning, or use four metal skewers.

2. Alternate the chicken cubes, tomatoes, and mushroom halves on skewers. Repeat until the skewers are full.

3. Combine the garlic, lemon zest and juice, olive oil, and oregano in a bowl. Put the skewers into a large dish and pour the marinade over them, lightly turning to coat. Marinate, refrigerated, for at least 2 hours or overnight. Preheat a charcoal grill, if using.

4. Place the skewers on a gas or charcoal grill and cook, rolling the skewers around every 3 to 4 minutes to ensure even cooking, until lightly seared, 12 to 14 minutes. Serve over salad.

SOUPS

SEAFOOD GUMBO

1.8 teaspoons sugar
1 hour to prepare and cook
Serves 8

1 tablespoon coconut oil

2 cups chopped onions

2 cups chopped celery

1 cup chopped green bell pepper

1 cup chopped red bell pepper

3 garlic cloves, minced

1 tablespoon Cajun seasoning mix or Creole spice blend

2 bay leaves

6 cups vegetable or chicken stock

One 14.5-ounce can chopped tomatoes

1 pound medium shrimp (30 count), peeled and deveined

1 cup lump crab meat

2 tablespoons hot sauce

1 cup sliced fresh or frozen okra (optional)

1. Heat the oil in a heavy-bottomed 5-quart saucepan over medium heat. Add the onions, celery, bell peppers, garlic, Cajun seasoning, and bay leaves. Sauté for 5 to 7 minutes, until the onions and peppers are softened.

2. Add the stock and tomatoes with their juices and bring to a boil. Reduce the heat and simmer for 40 minutes.

3. Add the shrimp, crab, hot sauce, and okra, if using. Return the mixture to a boil, cover, and remove from the heat; let stand for 10

minutes or until the shrimp turn pink. Remove the bay leaves before serving.

BUTTERNUT CHOWDER

2.6 teaspoons sugar
1 hour to prepare and cook
Serves 4

2 teaspoons coconut oil
1 cup shelled unsalted pumpkin seeds (pepitas)
2 pounds butternut squash, peeled and cut into 1-inch cubes
8 cups vegetable stock
1 large tomato, chopped
1 onion, chopped
1 green bell pepper, chopped
1 jalapeño pepper or Scotch Bonnet chile, seeded and minced
    (optional)
1 tablespoon minced fresh ginger
8 scallions, green and white parts chopped
3 sprigs fresh thyme, stems removed
¼ cup chopped fresh cilantro, plus cilantro sprigs for garnish
Juice from 1 lime

1. Heat the oil in a small skillet over medium heat. Add the pumpkin seeds and toast, stirring frequently, until they begin to brown and pop, 5 to 7 minutes. Remove from the heat and set aside.

2. Combine the squash, stock, tomato, onion, bell pepper, chile, ginger, scallions, and thyme in a large pot. Place over high heat and simmer uncovered for about 45 minutes, stirring occasionally, until the vegetables are tender.

3. Remove from the heat and blend with an immersion blender for 2 to 4 minutes, until smooth. Add the cilantro and lime juice. Serve with a sprinkling of pepitas and a sprig of cilantro.

VEGETABLE SOUP

1.6 teaspoons sugar
1 hour to prepare and cook
Serves 8

2 tablespoons coconut oil

2 cups chopped onion

5 garlic cloves, minced

2 ribs celery, chopped

1 cup sliced green beans (in 2-inch pieces)

½ cup sliced carrot (in ¼-inch pieces)

1 zucchini, halved lengthwise and sliced

5 fresh basil leaves

1 teaspoon dried oregano

1 teaspoon dried rosemary

4 cups vegetable broth

4 cups purified water

One 15-ounce can light kidney beans, drained

Two 16-ounce cans chopped tomatoes

2 cups shredded green cabbage

1 teaspoons salt

1 teaspoon freshly ground black pepper

1. Heat the oil in a stockpot over medium-high heat. Add the onion and garlic, and sauté for 2 minutes.

2. Stir in the celery, vegetables, and herbs. Add the broth, water, beans, and tomatoes. Bring to a boil, reduce the heat, and simmer for 30 minutes.

3. Add the cabbage, salt, and pepper; cook 5 minutes more, until the cabbage wilts. Serve.

TOMATO BASIL SOUP

1.6 teaspoons sugar
1 hour to prepare and cook
Serves 8

> 4 cups chopped, seeded, peeled ripe tomato
> 4 cups tomato juice
> ⅓ cup fresh basil leaves
> 1 cup chicken stock
> ¼ teaspoon salt
> ¼ teaspoon freshly ground black pepper
> ½ cup plain yogurt

1. Bring the tomatoes and tomato juice to a boil in a large saucepan. Reduce the heat and simmer uncovered for 30 minutes.

2. Place the tomato mixture and basil (reserving a few leaves for garnish) in a blender or food processor and process until smooth. Return the pureed mixture to the pan. Add the chicken stock, salt, and pepper.

3. Add the yogurt, stirring with a whisk. Cook over medium heat until thickened, about 5 minutes more. Serve the soup garnished with a few basil leaves.

MAINS

EGGPLANT ROULADES

4.2 teaspoons sugar
1 hour to prepare and cook
Serves 6

> 2 medium eggplants
> 2 teaspoons extra-virgin olive oil
> One 15-ounce container ricotta
> ½ cup grated Parmesan cheese

½ cup shredded mozzarella cheese

1 large egg, lightly beaten

1 cup fresh spinach leaves

¼ cup fresh basil leaves

2 cups tomato puree (or 3 medium tomatoes, pulsed in a food processor)

1. Preheat the oven to 375°F. Slice the eggplant lengthwise into pieces about ¼-inch thick. Put the eggplant in a baking pan and coat lightly on both sides with the olive oil. Bake until slices are lightly softened and flexible, about 5 to 6 minutes. Cool to room temperature. Keep the oven on.

2. Combine the ricotta, ¼ cup of the Parmesan, ¼ cup of the mozzarella, the egg, spinach, and basil in a food processor with a standard S blade, or mix by hand with a whisk in a large mixing bowl (chop the spinach first, if working by hand).

3. Pour half of the tomato puree in the bottom of a 9 x 12-inch baking dish. Place a large spoonful of the cheese mixture on the end of each slice of eggplant and roll it up. Place the rolled eggplant in the pan, seam side down, then cover with the remaining tomato puree and sprinkle the top with the remaining Parmesan and mozzarella cheeses.

4. Cover with a lid or foil and bake for 25 to 30 minutes, until the eggplant rolls are heated through. Remove the lid and bake for an additional 5 to 10 minutes, until the cheese begins to brown. Let stand for 5 to 10 minutes before serving.

GROUPER-N-GREENS

1.6 teaspoons sugar
20 minutes to prepare and cook
Serves 4

2 tablespoons coconut oil
4 cups chopped trimmed kale or chard
1 shallot, thinly sliced
3 garlic cloves, sliced
2 tablespoons water
Two 8-ounce grouper fillets (or other white fish)
Salt and freshly ground black pepper
Juice of 1 lemon
4 fresh chives, thinly sliced

1. Heat 1 tablespoon of the coconut oil in a large sauté pan over medium heat. Add the kale, shallot, and garlic and sauté, stirring occasionally, until the vegetables are slightly softened, about 5 to 7 minutes. Add the water, cover, and steam for about 1 minute, until the water has cooked off. Remove greens from the pan and set aside.

2. Wipe out the pan with a paper towel and reheat with the remaining 1 tablespoon coconut oil over medium-high heat. Season the fish with salt and pepper, and place it in the pan, skin side down if there's skin. Cook for 5 to 6 minutes, until lightly browned and crisp on the bottom. Turn over and cook for another 4 minutes.

3. Serve the fish, cut in half, over the greens; sprinkle with lemon juice and garnish with the chives.

BAKED FISH

1.4 teaspoons sugar
15 minutes to prepare and cook
Serves 2

Two 4-ounce fish fillets, any variety of white fish
One 10-ounce package fresh spinach

2 small plum tomatoes, sliced
2 shallots, thinly sliced
1 tablespoon chopped pitted black olives
1 tablespoon drained capers
2 tablespoons fresh orange juice
Freshly ground black pepper

1. Preheat the oven to 400°F. Place the fillets in a shallow glass baking dish. Top with the spinach, tomatoes, shallots, olives, and capers. Drizzle the orange juice over the assembly.

2. Bake the fish for about 10 minutes per inch of thickness. Sprinkle the fish with the pepper and serve immediately, with vegetables or salad.

GRILLED MAHI MAHI WITH SPINACH

0.8 teaspoon sugar
30 minutes to prepare and cook
Serves 2

Two 4-ounce mahi mahi steaks
2 teaspoons coconut oil
1 shallot
2 garlic cloves
Salt and freshly ground black pepper
2 large tomatoes, peeled, seeded, and chopped
2 cups spinach leaves
Juice of 1 lime

1. Prepare a grill. Rinse the fish steaks and pat dry. Brush with some of the coconut oil and grill over medium heat, about 8 minutes per side or until the fish becomes flakey.

2. While the fish is grilling, use the remaining coconut oil to coat the bottom of a skillet. Sauté the shallot and garlic until the shallot is tender, 2 to 3 minutes. Sprinkle with salt and pepper.

3. Add the tomatoes and spinach, and cook, stirring, until the spinach starts to wilt, another 2 to 3 minutes.

4. Place the spinach mixture on top of the fish steaks. Sprinkle with the lime juice and serve.

GRILLED WILD SALMON WITH MANGO RELISH

2.2 teaspoons sugar
20 minutes to prepare and cook
Serves 2

Relish

½ small mango, pulp scooped out and diced

2 tablespoons diced red bell pepper

1 tablespoon diced red onion

1 tablespoon chopped fresh parsley

1 tablespoon chopped fresh cilantro

1 teaspoon grated lime zest

½ tablespoon minced garlic

1 teaspoon fresh lime juice

Fish

Two 4-ounce pieces wild salmon fillet

Salt and freshly ground black pepper

1. For the relish: Combine all the ingredients and chill in the refrigerator for 1 hour. Heat a charcoal grill, if using.

2. For the fish: Season the fillets with salt and pepper and grill until the fish flakes, about 4 minutes per side.

3. Top the salmon with the relish and serve with vegetables or salad.

WILD SALMON WITH CITRUS MARINADE

2.2 teaspoons sugar
15 minutes to prepare and cook, 1 to 2 hours to marinate
Serves 2

¼ cup balsamic vinegar

¼ cup fresh orange juice

¼ cup fresh lemon or lime juice

2 teaspoons spicy brown mustard

Two 4-ounce pieces wild salmon fillet

1. Whisk the vinegar, orange and lemon or lime juices, and mustard in a bowl. Add the salmon and coat well to marinate. Place in the refrigerator for 1 to 2 hours. Preheat a charcoal grill, if using.

2. Remove the salmon from the marinade and place on a hot grill, skin side up, for 2 minutes. Turn the salmon skin side down and use the marinade to baste while cooking for 4 to 5 more minutes, until the salmon turns pale pink or flakes with a fork.

3. Serve the salmon with vegetables or salad.

THYME-STUFFED STEAK ON CRESS

1.4 teaspoons sugar
30 minutes to prepare and cook
Serves 2

8 ounces lean boneless beef (top round or sirloin)

2 teaspoons coconut oil

1 medium sweet onion, thinly sliced

Leaves from 2 sprigs fresh thyme

1 cup watercress leaves, stems removed

½ teaspoon cracked black peppercorns

1 tablespoon balsamic vinegar

2 cups watercress

1. Cut the beef into two equal portions crosswise, then slice a pocket into one side of each portion. Set aside.

2. Heat the oil in a large sauté pan over medium-high heat. Add the onion and sauté for 4 to 6 minutes, stirring occasionally, until the onion is well browned and tender. Add the thyme and watercress leaves during the last minute. When the filling is cool enough to handle, stuff the steaks with the onion mixture, securing the flaps with a toothpick. Season the steaks with the peppercorns, pressing so they adhere.

3. Preheat a stovetop grill pan over medium-high heat. Place the stuffed steaks on the grill pan and cook until browned on both sides, about 3 to 4 minutes per side. Remove from the heat and let rest for 3 to 5 minutes.

4. Drizzle the steaks with the balsamic vinegar and serve over a bed of watercress.

PERSIAN KEBABS

0.8 teaspoons sugar
30 minutes to prepare and cook
Serves 4

1 pound lean boneless beef (top round or sirloin), cubed
1 large onion, quartered and thickly sliced
4 firm plum tomatoes, thickly sliced
½ teaspoon salt
½ teaspoon lemon pepper
1 tablespoon sumac (optional)
1 teaspoon coconut oil
1 cup raw spinach leaves

1. Arrange the beef cubes, onion, and tomatoes on four skewers. Season the skewers overall with the salt, lemon pepper, and sumac, if using.

2. Coat a stovetop grill pan with the coconut oil and heat over medium-high heat. Add the skewers and cook, rotating occasionally, for 4 to 6 minutes per side.

3. Serve the skewers on a bed of raw spinach.

MEAT AND VEGGIE BOLOGNESE

2.2 teaspoons sugar
1 hour to prepare and cook
Serves 6

2 teaspoons coconut oil

1½ pounds lean ground beef (sirloin or top round)

1 onion, chopped

2 ribs celery, chopped

1 carrot, chopped

1 cup button mushrooms, chopped

3 garlic cloves, minced

1 tablespoon fresh oregano leaves

2 bay leaves

Two 28-ounce cans chopped tomatoes

½ cup fresh basil leaves, cut into chiffonade (rolled and sliced)

1. Heat the oil in a large heavy-bottomed pot over medium heat. Add the ground beef and cook 3 to 4 minutes, until lightly browned. Drain off all excess fat, leaving the meat in the pan. Then add the onion, celery, carrot, mushrooms, garlic, oregano, and bay leaves and sauté for 3 to 4 minutes.

2. Add the tomatoes with their juices and bring to a boil. Reduce the heat, cover, and simmer for 45 minutes. Remove the bay leaves.

3. Serve over Spaghetti Squash "Pasta" (page 221) topped with the basil.

SICILIAN CITRUS PORK

0.6 teaspoon sugar
1 hour to prepare and cook, 1+ hours to marinate
Serves 6

One 2-pound center-cut boneless pork roast, surface scored with a
   knife
2 garlic cloves, minced
1 teaspoon fennel seeds, crushed
½ teaspoon cumin seeds, crushed
1 tablespoon minced fresh rosemary leaves
½ teaspoon crushed black peppercorns
1 tablespoon olive oil
1 orange, cut into thin slices
½ cup water

1. Cover the scored top of the pork roast with the garlic, fennel, cumin, rosemary, and peppercorns; brush lightly with the oil and
then rub gently with the herbs. Transfer the pork to a zippered plastic
bag and add the orange slices. Seal tightly and marinate for at least 1
hour or overnight in the refrigerator.

2. Preheat the oven to 375°F. Remove the pork and orange slices
from the bag and place in a roasting pan. Add the water and cover the
pan with a lid or foil; roast for about 40 minutes.

3. Remove the lid and continue to roast the pork for about 15
minutes more, basting occasionally with the pan juices, until the internal temperature reads 160°F on a meat thermometer. Slice and
serve the meat with vegetables or salad.

LEMONGRASS CHICKEN

1.6 teaspoons sugar
25 minutes to prepare and cook, 1+ hours to marinate
Serves 4

3 garlic cloves, minced

1 large shallot, minced

1 tablespoon curry powder

1 fresh chile, such as serrano or jalapeño, seeds removed, flesh
    minced

2 fresh lemongrass stalks, outer layers removed, minced

1½ pounds boneless, skinless chicken breast, cut into 2-inch chunks

1 tablespoon tamari

1 tablespoon coconut oil

2 tablespoons water

1 tablespoon minced fresh ginger

1 bunch (about 1 pound) Swiss chard, trimmed and chopped

4 scallions, green and white parts thinly sliced

1. In a medium bowl, combine the garlic, shallot, curry powder, chile, and lemongrass. Add the chicken and tamari and stir to coat well. Marinate in the refrigerator for at least 1 hour.

2. Heat ½ tablespoon of the oil in a large sauté pan or wok over high heat. Add the marinated chicken and stir-fry, turning every few minutes, until well browned on all sides, about 8 minutes. Add the water and continue to cook until the chicken is fragrant, appears glazed, and is cooked through when pierced with a fork or knife, about 5 minutes more. Remove from the pan and set aside.

3. Wipe out the pan with a paper towel and heat the remaining ½ tablespoon oil in the same pan. Add the ginger and stir-fry for 1 minute. Add the chard and stir-fry for 2 minutes, or until the chard is wilted and the ginger is fragrant.

4. Place the chard on a serving plate and top with the chicken pieces. Serve garnished with the scallions.

CHICKEN MILANESE

1.2 teaspoons sugar
30 minutes to prepare and cook
Serves 2

One 8-ounce boneless, skinless chicken breast, cut in half
½ cup chickpea flour
1 tablespoon minced fresh parsley
1 teaspoon Italian seasoning
¼ teaspoon red pepper flakes
2 large egg whites, lightly beaten
2 tablespoons olive oil
2 cups loosely packed baby arugula
¼ red onion, thinly sliced
Juice of 1 lemon
1 tablespoon shavings Parmesan cheese

1. Place the chicken breast halves between sheets of wax paper or plastic wrap and lightly flatten with a meat mallet or rolling pin. Preheat the oven to 375°F.

2. In a low, flat bowl or pie pan, combine the chickpea flour, parsley, Italian seasoning, and red pepper flakes. Place the egg whites in a medium bowl. Moisten the chicken breasts in the egg whites, then dredge in the chickpea flour mixture, covering well.

3. Heat 1 tablespoon of the olive oil in a large ovenproof skillet over medium-high heat. Place the chicken breasts in the skillet and cook for 3 to 5 minutes per side, until golden. If necessary, transfer the pan with the chicken to the oven to cook an additional 5 to 10 minutes per side, until the chicken reaches an internal temperature of 160°F.

4. Serve the chicken breasts over the arugula and red onion slices. Drizzle the remaining 1 tablespoon olive oil and the lemon juice on top and sprinkle with the Parmesan shavings.

ZESTY CHICKEN PATTIES

1 teaspoon sugar
50 minutes to prepare, chill, and cook
Serves 2

½ pound ground chicken
2 shallots, chopped
2 tablespoons chopped fresh cilantro
1 garlic clove, minced
½ teaspoon cayenne
1 egg white, lightly beaten
Salt and freshly ground pepper
½ tablespoon coconut oil
1 lemon, halved

1. Mix all ingredients except the coconut oil and lemon in a bowl. Shape the mixture into two patties and chill for 30 minutes to set.

2. Heat the coconut oil in a sauté pan and cook the patties over medium heat, about 4 minutes per side or until done.

3. Squeeze the lemon over the patties and serve with salad greens.

CHICKEN IN A LETTUCE BOWL

1 teaspoon sugar
15 minutes to prepare and cook
Serves 2

1 tablespoon coconut oil

8 ounces ground chicken

1 garlic clove

½ can water chestnuts, drained and chopped

½ tablespoon oyster sauce

1½ teaspoons tamari

2 scallions, green and white parts chopped

2 whole Bibb lettuce leaves

1. Heat a large wok or frying pan over high heat. Add the oil and swirl to coat the pan. Add the chicken and garlic and stir-fry for 6 to 8 minutes, until the chicken is cooked through. Keep the mixture loose. Pour off any excess liquid.

2. Turn down the heat and add the water chestnuts, oyster sauce, tamari, and scallions.

3. Trim the lettuce leaves to form two lettuce cups. Divide the mixture between them and serve.

ASIAN CHICKEN WITH BOK CHOY

2.2 teaspoons sugar
40 minutes to prepare and cook, 2 hours to marinate
Serves 2

1 tablespoon tamari
1 tablespoon rice wine vinegar
½ teaspoon dark sesame oil
½ tablespoon grated fresh ginger
2 boneless, skinless chicken breast halves
½ pound bok choy, trimmed
5 dried shiitake mushrooms
¼ cup chicken stock
½ tablespoon cornstarch

1. Combine the tamari, vinegar, sesame oil, and ginger in a bowl. Add the chicken to a zippered plastic bag and pour in the marinade. Shake to cover, and marinate for at least 2 hours. When ready to cook, remove the chicken and reserve the marinade.

2. Put the chicken in a bamboo steamer basket set over boiling water in a medium saucepan. Cover and steam for 6 minutes. Turn the chicken over and steam for an additional 6 minutes. Place the bok choy on top of the chicken and continue steaming until the chicken is done and the bok choy is tender, about 5 minutes more.

3. Place the reserved marinade and the mushrooms in a saucepan over medium heat. Simmer until the mushrooms are tender, about 5 minutes.

4. In small bowl, add enough of the stock to the cornstarch to make a paste. Add the paste and remaining stock to the mushroom marinade and continue simmering until the sauce thickens, an additional 2 to 3 minutes.

5. Assemble the bok choy and chicken on plates, drizzle the sauce over, and serve.

CHICKEN MARSALA

2.6 teaspoons sugar
30 minutes to prepare and cook
Serves 2

 2 boneless, skinless chicken breast halves
 1 tablespoon rice flour
 ¼ teaspoon salt
 ¼ teaspoon freshly ground black pepper
 ½ teaspoon coconut oil
 ¼ cup sliced mushrooms
 ¼ cup marsala wine
 ¼ cup chicken broth
 1 tablespoon fresh lemon juice
 ½ tablespoon chopped fresh flat parsley

1. Place the chicken breast halves between sheets of wax paper or plastic wrap and lightly flatten with a meat mallet or rolling pin. Mix the flour, salt, and pepper, and then dredge the chicken in the flour mixture. Shake off the excess.

2. Heat the oil in a large sauté pan over medium-high heat. Add the chicken and brown on each side, about 3 minutes per side. Remove the chicken and set aside.

3. Add the mushrooms, wine, broth, and lemon juice and simmer for 10 minutes or until the mixture is reduced to ⅓ cup.

4. Return the chicken to the pan, turning to coat well. Cover and cook until the chicken is cooked through, about 5 minutes. Sprinkle with parsley and serve.

CHICKEN ASPARAGUS STIR-FRY

1.4 teaspoons sugar
25 minutes to prepare and cook
Serves 2

1 tablespoon coconut oil
1 garlic clove, minced
1 tablespoon minced fresh ginger
One 8-ounce boneless, skinless chicken breast, sliced
1 minced shallot
¾ cup fresh asparagus, trimmed and sliced
2 tablespoons tamari
¼ cup water
2 ounces slivered almonds

1. Heat a large sauté pan or wok over high heat. Add the oil and swirl to coat. Add the garlic, ginger, and chicken and stir-fry for 1 to 2 minutes, until the chicken turns white.

2. Add the shallot and asparagus and stir-fry for 2 more minutes. Reduce the heat and simmer for 2 more minutes.

3. Stir in the tamari and water. Cover and continue to simmer for 2 more minutes, until the chicken is cooked through and the asparagus is tender but still firm, 1 to 2 minutes more. Toss in the almonds, stir quickly, and serve.

LIGURIAN CHICKEN

3.6 teaspoons sugar
1 hour to prepare and cook
Serves 4

1 cup cooked chickpeas
1 tablespoon coconut oil
3 cups chopped kale leaves
2 garlic cloves, minced
4 scallions, green and white parts minced
2 tablespoons grated Parmesan cheese
1 large onion, sliced
1 large ripe tomato, chopped
Leaves from 1 bunch fresh mint
Four 6-ounce boneless, skinless chicken breast halves, pounded lightly
1 lemon, sliced
½ teaspoon red pepper flakes
2 cups water or chicken stock

1. Preheat the oven to 400°F. In a medium bowl, lightly mash the chickpeas with a fork.

2. Heat the oil in a large sauté pan over medium-high heat. Add the kale and garlic and sauté for 2 minutes. Add the chickpeas, and then stir in the scallions and cheese. Let cool.

3. Scatter the onion and tomato on the bottom of a 9 x 12-inch baking dish. Layer in the mint leaves.

4. Gently fold the chicken breasts around the chickpea mixture and add the chicken "packages" to the baking dish. Top with the lemon slices and red pepper flakes and pour the stock around the chicken.

5. Lightly cover the pan with a lid or foil and bake for 30 to 35 minutes. Remove the lid and bake for an additional 10 to 15 minutes, until the chicken breasts are cooked through. Serve with the pan juices.

UNSTUFFED CABBAGE

3.4 teaspoons sugar
1 hour to prepare and cook
Serves 4

2 teaspoons coconut oil

1 medium onion, chopped

2 small carrots, shredded

1 pound lean ground turkey

4 cups shredded green cabbage

One 28-ounce can chopped tomatoes

1 cup tomato puree

¼ cup apple cider vinegar

1. Heat the oil in a large skillet over medium heat. Add the onion and carrots and sauté for 5 minutes. Add the onion and carrots and sauté for 5 minutes. Add the turkey and sauté for 5 minutes, then add the cabbage and sauté for 2 minutes more.

2. Add the tomatoes with their juices, tomato puree, and vinegar. Bring to a boil, then reduce the heat, cover, and simmer for 45 minutes. Serve in bowls.

TURKEY BURGERS

1.4 teaspoons sugar
30 minutes to prepare and cook
Serves 2

½ pound ground turkey breast

1 garlic clove, minced

½ teaspoon Cajun seasoning

Dash of freshly ground black pepper

2 tablespoons light teriyaki sauce

1 onion, sliced ¼ inch thick

2 teaspoons coconut oil

1. Combine the turkey, garlic, seasoning, pepper, and teriyaki sauce in a large bowl. Divide the mixture into two patties.

2. Put 1 teaspoon of the coconut oil in a sauté pan and cook over medium heat. Add the onion slices and sauté until they are tender and brown, about 5 minutes. Remove the onion from the pan and set aside.

3. Add the remaining 1 teaspoon coconut oil to the pan and add the patties. Cook for 5 to 10 minutes over medium heat, turning to brown both sides, until the patties are cooked through.

4. Place a turkey patty on each plate and top with the onion slices. Serve over mixed salad greens.

TURKEY ROLL WITH GOAT CHEESE AND SPINACH

3.4 teaspoons sugar
1 hour 15 minutes to prepare and cook
Serves 4

One 1-pound boneless, skinless turkey breast
Salt
1 sweet potato, peeled and thinly sliced
1 cup baby spinach leaves
¼ cup frozen unsweetened cherries
¼ cup pecans, chopped
2 garlic cloves, minced
¼ cup goat cheese, crumbled
2 tablespoons rice flour
1 teaspoon coconut oil
Freshly ground black pepper

1. Preheat the oven to 375°F. Place the turkey between sheets of wax paper or plastic wrap and lightly flatten with a meat mallet or rolling pin. Salt it lightly.

2. Layer the sweet potato slices, spinach, cherries, pecans, garlic, and goat cheese onto the turkey cutlet. Roll up tightly, tie with string, and dust with rice flour.

3. Coat an ovenproof skillet with the coconut oil, heat to medium, add the turkey roll, and brown on all sides. Cover the skillet and place in the oven. Bake the turkey roll for 30 to 45 minutes, or until cooked through.

4. Let the turkey roll rest for 10 minutes before slicing, and serve either plain or with your choice of vegetables.

SIDES

HOMEMADE SAUERKRAUT (FERMENTED VEGETABLES)

0.8 teaspoon sugar
30 minutes to prepare, 7+ days to ferment
Serves 16

    5 tablespoons fine sea salt
    1 quart purified water
    2 heads red and/or green cabbage, cored and shredded

1. Combine 3 tablespoons of the salt and the water in a large bowl. Let sit until the salt dissolves completely. (Or, add the salt to 2 pints warm purified water, stir, then add the remaining 2 pints cold water.)

2. Place the cabbage in a large bowl and sprinkle evenly with 1 tablespoon salt. Massage and squeeze the cabbage thoroughly with your hands so that the natural juices of the cabbage are released into the bowl.

3. Transfer the cabbage and juices to ten 12-ounce wide-mouth glass jars or a 1-gallon crock, pressing it down tightly. Sprinkle with the remaining 1 tablespoon salt. The juices may completely cover the cabbage. If not, add brine to submerge the cabbage in the liquid. The liquid should be no closer than 1 inch from the lid. If the cabbage floats above the liquid, you will need to weigh it down with a plate or lid.

4. Leave the jars or crock in a dark, warm place in your kitchen, such as a pantry or cabinet. Allow the cabbage to ferment for at least

7 days, loosening and retightening the lid, if you are using a jar, every 3 days to release pressure. Check regularly to be sure the cabbage remains submerged, adding more brine if necessary.

5. After 7 days, taste the sauerkraut. If it is not yet to your liking, wait another day and taste again, and so on, until it reaches the desired flavor.

6. Move the jar to the refrigerator to slow any further fermentation and to set the flavor. If you've used a large crock, portion the sauerkraut into jars or glass storage containers to store in the refrigerator.

WARM 'SHROOMS-N-SPINACH

2.2 teaspoons sugar
15 minutes to prepare and cook
Serves 4

2 tablespoons white miso
2 tablespoons rice vinegar (sugar-free)
1 tablespoon coconut oil
1 cup sliced button mushrooms
1 cup sliced shiitake mushroom caps
1 cup sliced cremini (baby bella) mushrooms
1 large shallot, minced (optional)
One 14-ounce package spinach leaves or baby spinach
2 tablespoons sliced almonds

1. In a small bowl, whisk the miso with the vinegar.

2. Heat half of the oil in a large skillet over medium-high heat. Add half of the mushrooms and shallot and sauté for 3 minutes, or until the mushrooms begin to brown. Remove from the heat and sauté the remaining mushrooms. Add all the mushrooms back to the pan. Pour the miso mixture over the mushrooms and cook for an additional minute.

3. Place the spinach in a serving bowl. Pour the mushroom mixture over the spinach, add the almonds, and toss. Serve warm.

INDIAN SPICED GARBANZOS

3.5 teaspoons sugar
25 minutes to prepare and cook
Serves 4

2 teaspoons coconut oil
½ onion, diced
1 tablespoon garam masala (or high-quality curry powder)
2 tablespoons tomato paste
One 15-ounce can chickpeas, drained and rinsed
1 cup cauliflower florets
One 14-ounce can vegetable stock
¼ cup fresh cilantro leaves, chopped
¼ cup plain Greek yogurt

1. Heat the oil in a large saucepan over medium-high heat. Add the onion and garam masala and sauté until the onion is softened and the seasonings are aromatic, 2 to 3 minutes. Add the tomato paste and sauté for 1 minute.

2. Add the chickpeas, cauliflower, and vegetable stock. Bring to a boil, then lower the heat and simmer until the cauliflower is tender, 10 to 12 minutes. If the liquid appears too thick, add a little water or additional vegetable stock.

3. Garnish each serving with the cilantro and a dollop of yogurt.

CAULIFLOWER "RICE" PILAF

0.6 teaspoon sugar
30 minutes to prepare and cook
Serves 8

1 head of cauliflower, core removed
2 tablespoons coconut oil
2 tablespoons chopped onion
2 ribs celery, chopped
1 garlic clove, minced
½ cup chicken broth
¼ teaspoon fennel seeds
¼ teaspoon dried oregano
Dash of curry powder
¼ cup slivered almonds, toasted

1. Grate the cauliflower using a cheese grater or food processor fitted with the grating blade.

2. Heat the coconut oil in a large sauté pan over medium heat. Add the onion, celery, garlic, and cauliflower. Sauté for 2 minutes.

3. Add the broth and spices. Sauté about 10 minutes more. Remove the pan from the heat. Stir in the toasted almonds and serve.

ROASTED BROCCOLI WITH LEMON AND SHALLOTS

2.1 teaspoons sugar
20 minutes to prepare and cook
Serves 2

2 cups broccoli florets
½ cup finely sliced shallots
1 teaspoon olive oil
Salt and freshly ground black pepper
Juice of ½ small lemon

1. Preheat the oven to 450°F. Toss the broccoli with the shallots, oil, salt, and pepper.

2. Spread the broccoli on a large baking sheet (with sides) and roast until the broccoli is tender and browned on the bottom, 10 to 12 minutes. Remove from the oven and sprinkle with the lemon juice. Toss gently and serve.

SPAGHETTI SQUASH "PASTA"

1.6 teaspoons sugar
40 minutes to prepare and cook
Serves 4

1 spaghetti squash
Salt and freshly ground black pepper

1. Preheat the oven to 400°F. Cut the squash in half lengthwise. Remove the seeds. Place the halves facedown in a baking dish; put about ½ inch of water in the bottom of the dish. Place the dish in the oven and bake for 30 minutes, or until tender.

2. When the squash has cooled a bit, turn the halves over. Using the prongs of a fork, scrape out the squash pulp. It will be stringlike. Season with salt and pepper to taste and serve as a side to replace pasta.

HOMEMADE SALSA IN AN AVOCADO BOAT

0.9 teaspoon sugar
30 minutes to prepare
Serves 2

2 large tomatoes, seeded and chopped
1 serrano chile or jalapeño pepper, chopped
⅓ cup chopped green and white parts of scallions
2 tablespoons chopped fresh cilantro
2 tablespoons fresh lime juice
¼ teaspoon salt
1 avocado, cut in half, seed removed, and partially hollowed out

Place all the ingredients except the avocado in a bowl and mix well. Chill for 20 minutes. Serve inside the partially hollowed-out avocado halves.

SPICY SAUTÉED KALE

2.8 teaspoons sugar
20 minutes to prepare and cook
Serves 6

1 tablespoon coconut oil
2 teaspoons minced garlic
½ cup chicken stock
1 large bunch kale, stemmed, leaves coarsely chopped
¼ teaspoon red pepper flakes
Freshly ground black pepper

1. Heat the oil in a deep skillet over medium heat. Add the garlic and stock; stir. Add the kale by handfuls, stirring to make room for more leaves as it shrinks in cooking.

2. Cover with a lid and cook, stirring occasionally, for 10 to 15 minutes, or until tender.

3. Add the red pepper flakes and black pepper to taste.

WILTED CABBAGE

0.6 teaspoon sugar
20 minutes to prepare and cook
Serves 6

1 teaspoon coconut oil
6 cups chopped green cabbage or Napa cabbage
¼ cup chicken stock
Freshly ground black pepper
½ teaspoon cumin seeds
2 teaspoons apple cider vinegar

1. Heat the oil in a Dutch oven or large pot over medium heat. Add the cabbage and stock and simmer, stirring occasionally, until the cabbage starts to wilt, 3 to 4 minutes. Stir in the pepper.

2. Put the cumin seeds in a small saucepan and toast over medium heat for 1 minute, shaking the pan frequently.

3. Add the toasted seeds and apple cider vinegar to the cabbage and cook for 15 more minutes, stirring occasionally, until tender.

"SWEET" SNACKS

BERRIES-N-CREAM

2.1 teaspoons sugar
5 minutes to prepare
Serves 1

One 6-ounce container plain Greek yogurt
4 tablespoons whipped cream
½ cup mixed berries (blueberries, strawberries, blackberries)
Mint leaf, for garnish

Combine the yogurt and whipped cream. Stir in the berries. Garnish with mint, if desired.

JOEL AND SANDI'S NUT BUTTER CHOCOLATE CUPS

0.2 teaspoon sugar
15 minutes to prepare, 25 minutes to chill
Serves 16, 2 cups per serving

   5 tablespoons coconut cream concentrate (coconut butter)
   5 tablespoons coconut oil (best if in liquid form)
   6 tablespoons cacao powder (see Note)
   1 tablespoon ground cinnamon
   1 teaspoon vanilla extract
   1 teaspoon lo han (monk fruit) sweetener
   3 tablespoons nut butter of choice (cashew, sunflower, almond)

1. Mix all the ingredients in a bowl except for the nut butter. Put
½ teaspoon of the mixture into each cup of a mini muffin pan. Freeze
for about 10 minutes. Set the remaining mixture aside.

2. Add ¼ teaspoon nut butter on top of each frozen "cup." Add
another ½ teaspoon of the cacao mixture on top of the nut butter,
then freeze again for about 15 minutes to harden.

Note: *Cacao powder is a less-processed version of cocoa powder and is
available at health food stores.*

JOY'S LEMON BLISS

0.2 teaspoon sugar
5 minutes to prepare, 2 hours to chill
Serves 1

   1 cup unsweetened almond milk
   2 tablespoons chia seeds
   1 teaspoon ground cinnamon
   12 drops vanilla stevia
   1 teaspoon lemon extract

Mix all the ingredients in a medium bowl. Chill in the refrigerator for 2 hours. Serve cold.

CACAO, AVOCADO, AND CHIA MOUSSE

0.6 teaspoon sugar
15 minutes to prepare, 1 hour to chill
Serves 4

1 avocado
¼ cup cacao powder
1 teaspoon vanilla extract
½ cup unsweetened almond milk
2 tablespoons chia seeds

Place the avocado, vanilla, and almond milk in a food processor and process until smooth. Stir in the chia seeds. Transfer the mixture to a medium bowl and refrigerate for 1 hour. Scoop into individual bowls and serve chilled.

COCO-NUT PUDDING

0.6 teaspoon sugar
15 minutes to prepare, 1 hour to chill
Serves 4

½ cup almond butter
3 tablespoons almond flour
3 tablespoons unsweetened shredded coconut
1 teaspoon coconut oil
1 teaspoon ground cinnamon
6 to 8 drops vanilla stevia (optional)
3 tablespoons chia seeds

Place the almond butter, almond flour, coconut and coconut oil, cinnamon, and stevia, if using, in a food processor and process until smooth. Stir in the chia seeds, then transfer to a small bowl and refrigerate for 1 hour. Scoop into individual bowls and serve chilled.

KEFIR ICE CREAM

0.5 teaspoon sugar for vanilla
0.6 teaspoon sugar for chocolate
0.7 teaspoon sugar for strawberry
15 minutes to prepare, 1 hour to chill
Serves 12 (1½ quarts ice cream)

2 large eggs
¼ cup lo han (monk fruit) sweetener or ¾ teaspoon stevia liquid
   (flavored, if desired)
2 cups kefir
1 cup heavy cream (or kefir cream made with heavy cream)
2 teaspoons vanilla extract

For chocolate: ⅔ cup unsweetened cocoa powder
For strawberry: 1 cup crushed strawberries

1. Beat the eggs well and add the sweetener. Blend in the kefir, cream, and vanilla.

2. Add the cocoa powder or strawberries, if desired.

3. Transfer the mixture to an ice cream maker and follow the manufacturer's instructions to make the ice cream. Place in the freezer to harden.

Note: *This recipe contains raw eggs. Please be cautious when consuming raw eggs, as many eggs are contaminated with salmonella bacteria.*

Flavored stevia can be used to experiment with new flavors. See Resources, page 254, for examples.

Chapter 14

RESCUE KIT FOR SUCCESS

With any new change in life there are growing pains. Fortunately, the growing pains that accompany the Skinny Gut Diet are short-lived. The dietary changes you will be making are designed to support your transition from eating a diet high in carbohydrates (and likely low in vegetables) to one that focuses on nonstarchy vegetables and low-sugar fruits, healthy fats, proteins, nuts, and seeds. But you will inevitably come up against situations that test your resolve—and your creativity. This rescue kit will help you integrate the Skinny Gut Diet anywhere, anyhow, so that you can stay on track moving toward your weight-loss goal.

HOW TO EAT OUT WITHOUT GIVING IN

If you are worried about what to eat when dining out, I'm here to allay your fears. Eating out is not as hard as you might think. Sure, you will not be eating the usual sandwich, pasta, or french fries, but there will always be options for you, no matter where you go. Read this section carefully so that you will be ready the next time you dine out.

A simple way to eat while dining out is the obvious: a salad with added protein in the form of grilled chicken, steak, fish, or shrimp. Most restaurants offer just such a salad. There are a few things to be careful about, however. You want to make sure that the added meat or seafood is not breaded. And ask them to hold the croutons or wonton strips.

Another great option is to order a tasty sandwich without the bun, along with a side salad. Instead of eating the side salad first, place the sandwich fillings (sans bun) on top of the salad and enjoy. Just be sure that the sandwich fillings you choose are not breaded. For example, maybe that chipotle chicken sandwich with Monterey Jack cheese looks good to you. Instead of lamenting the loss of sandwiches altogether, order the sandwich as I've suggested. Not only will you get a delicious meal, but you'll also have a healthy portion of fresh veggies in the salad. Bon appétit!

Yet another choice is to order a protein entrée along with vegetables as sides. Grilled steak, pork, chicken, fish, and shellfish are commonly offered as dinner entrées. Simply forgo the potatoes, french fries, rice, and other starchy options and instead fill your plate with greens or whatever nonstarchy vegetables they have to offer. Again, steer clear of breaded meats and seafood, as well as thick sauces to which flour has been added (this is more common than you think).

As you can see, dining out is not the carb trap you thought it would be. There will always be options; you simply need to know what to look for and when to be creative. Some restaurants are more amenable than others when it comes to variety, and sometimes they will forget and bring the bun anyway (set it aside—step away from the bun), but you will certainly be able to enjoy a delicious meal wherever you go.

DINNER PARTY TACTICS

The dreaded dinner party with your Italian in-laws—you know the scene: pasta galore, bread with every bite, sweet desserts to tempt even the most devout Skinny Gut Dieter. This may be the absolute worst-case scenario of dinner parties, so let's figure out how to get through it without gaining 10 pounds or alienating your loved ones, shall we? If you can do this, you can do anything.

First step: at least a few days (preferably a week) before the dinner party, call your hostess and let her know that you are on a diet that doesn't include breads, pastas, potatoes, or sweets. Let her know that you really appreciate all the work that goes into preparing such a feast, and that you would like to offer to bring something of your own. Ask her if there will be a protein (that's not smothered in pasta or bread crumbs), such as chicken or fish, that you could eat. If not, offer to bring something. Or, ask her if she minds if you bring your own low-carb pasta (see Resources, page 254, for excellent options). By connecting with the hostess ahead of time, your chances of being able to eat at the dinner party without pushing green beans across your plate and dodging awkward glances all night will be greatly improved. This call is vital to your success.

Next step: before you leave for the party, eat a small meal. Chances are there will be piles of delicious-looking food that may tempt your reserves. Going on a semi-full stomach will help you stay the course. You can do this. I believe in you. After you succeed, invite the attendees to a dinner party at *your* house. Show them that it can be easy and delicious to eat healthy while not feeling deprived. Perhaps as a result, the next dinner party will offer you more options.

ALWAYS HAVE A PLAN

It's important to think about the foods you will eat for the week coming up. I know I mentioned it earlier, but it bears repeating: *Have a plan.* By planning your days and weeks, you will be more likely to succeed. Take some time each weekend to think about your next week. What will you eat for breakfast? Lunch? Dinner? What about your snacks? How about dessert? Can you eat dinner leftovers for lunch the next day? Plan it. By making a plan you'll be less likely to find yourself hungry and with no good options. Don't leave yourself stranded. Take a few minutes each weekend to plan, and put that plan into action at the grocery store and in your kitchen.

I am a big fan of packing a cooler with snacks and lunch to keep me going throughout the day, as you learned in Chapter 10. Get in the habit of preparing your lunch and portioning your snacks the night before, so that you can pack your cooler and head out the door at your usual pace, prepared to eat for the day. This simple measure will go a long way toward your reaching your goal, especially if you work a nine-to-five job that leaves little time for cooking and eating.

DELICIOUS CARB SUBSTITUTES

When it comes to getting those carb treats you used to crave, you will be glad to hear that there are options for these foods that are Skinny Gut Diet–approved. One of the best ways to enjoy baked treats that are low in sugar is to use flours of almond and coconut. If you miss crunchy snacks like crackers, you can make crackers using these flours, too. If you miss the sweet treats, you can make cookies using these flours and substituting natural sweeteners such as stevia, erythritol, and lo han (monk fruit). See Resources, page 255, for a great website that offers delicious recipes. If you are not the baking type and you miss the crunch of crackers and chips, there are some crackers that you can eat *in moderation* that will allow you to get the crunchy mouth feel you love. (See Resources, page 254, for my recommendations.)

Finally, for the pasta lovers, I found the perfect low-carb pasta that tastes delicious. (See Resources, page 254, for my recommendations for all these foods and more.) Another option for pasta is to use a tool called a spiralizer, or spiral slicer, and make "pasta" out of raw zucchini. All you do is spiralize the zucchini and you have instant pasta. You can heat it briefly in a pan or serve it raw for a delicious and nutritious pasta substitute. Or, you can make pasta out of spaghetti squash (where do you think it got that name?). See the recipe for Spaghetti Squash "Pasta" (page 221).

GROCERY SHOPPING STRATEGY GUIDE

You will notice something very interesting after you have been on the Skinny Gut Diet for a few weeks. Your grocery shopping pattern will shift. Have you ever heard the advice to shop the perimeter of the grocery store for the healthiest foods? You will find that you naturally shop the perimeter when eating on the Skinny Gut Diet. For the most part, the aisles in the center of the store are filled with packaged, well-marketed, sugar- and carb-filled non-foods. You will want to steer clear of these aisles, with the exception of the occasional dash down the condiments and spices aisle or the coffee and tea aisle.

Fill your cart with plenty of nonstarchy vegetables, low-sugar fruits, proteins, healthy fats, nuts, and seeds. Your shopping cart will contain the foods you intend to eat while leaving behind the foods that tend to "jump" into your cart when you're not looking. You know what foods I mean: cookies, crackers, chips, doughnuts. Simply skip those aisles and stay focused on the course at hand—your skinny gut.

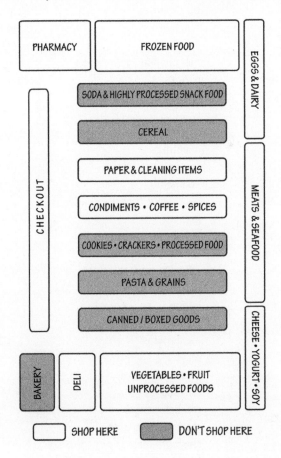

Shopping List

The following shopping list gives you an idea of what you will buy at the grocery store each week so that you can have everything you need to succeed on the Skinny Gut Diet. Please use this list as a suggestion to help guide your planning. Having a list on hand will help you to shop in an organized way, without getting distracted by foods you do not need. (See Resources, pages 253 to 254, for rescue foods such as low-carb pasta and crackers that you can enjoy.)

Proteins	Veggies & Fruits	Condiments
almond butter	avocados	apple cider vinegar
unsweetened nut milks	baby arugula	coconut oil
blue cheese crumbles	baby spinach	Dijon mustard
buttermilk	blackberries	extra-virgin olive oil
cannellini beans	blueberries	mayonnaise
Cheddar cheese	broccoli	mustard
chicken	can chopped tomatoes	pickle relish
chicken sausage	carrots	tamari
chicken stock	celery	
chicken tenderloins	chard	
chickpeas	cherry tomatoes	
cottage cheese	cilantro	
eggs	cucumber	
kefir	edamame	
lean ground beef	sauerkraut (non-pasteurized)	
mixed nuts	garlic	
Parmesan cheese	green bell pepper	
plain Greek yogurt	green cabbage	
pork roast	jalapeño pepper	
sunflower seeds	kale	
tahini	lemon	
turkey bacon	lime	
turkey jerky	mushrooms	
turkey slices	onions	
	parsley	
	pineapple	
	red bell pepper	
	roasted red peppers	
	salad greens	

Proteins	Veggies & Fruits	Condiments
	scallions	
	strawberries	
	tomatoes	
	tomato puree	
	zucchini	

HOW TO CHEAT WITHOUT HAVING TO START OVER

If you are surprised at the idea that I might let you cheat, rest assured that I have not lost my marbles. No one is perfect. There may come a time when you simply can't refuse that chocolate cake or Aunt Florence's lasagna. I understand. But I want you to succeed. You see, what tends to happen is that once we cheat one time, we figure that we may as well eat another piece of cake, since we're already cheating. And then once we're "officially cheating," we decide that we may as well eat all those foods we have been missing. The snowball effect is fierce when it comes to cheating on your diet. You know what I mean.

Instead, if you find yourself eating that piece of cake, or pizza, or french fries, let it be an isolated incident. Eat one serving—one *bite* if you can—and then move on. Be aware that your mind will try to play tricks on you, trying to convince you of why it would be a good idea to eat *more* of these foods. When this happens, picture the bad bacteria in your gut conspiring to get you to crave more carbs and sugars. They want that food even more than you do! And then reach for a high-protein snack to quell the cravings. The downside of cheating is that it often leads to binge-like behaviors that contribute to serious setbacks in progress, or even complete abandonment of the diet. If you tend to crave sweets, treat yourself to a dessert from Chapter 13. With a maximum of 2.1 teaspoons of sugar per serving, these treats will satisfy your sweet tooth without putting you over your sugar quota. If salty, crunchy snacks are your weakness, find some high-fiber, low-carb, gluten-free crackers and prepare five crackers topped with cheese. Put the box away. (This step is crucial.) Savor each bite.

And then move on. If you are craving more, eat a handful of nuts, a slice of deli meat, or a deviled egg. Problem solved.

EXERCISE

If you already have an exercise regimen in place before you start the Skinny Gut Diet, great—keep doing what you're doing. Exercise is an important component in a healthy lifestyle. But if you are not exercising regularly at the onset of this diet, wait until you get acclimated before adding any exercise. My reason for this is simple: I want you to succeed. If you take on too many new lifestyle changes at once, you are less likely to be successful at any of them. If you are not exercising now, save it for later. Once you have fully implemented this way of eating and you feel very comfortable with it, then go ahead and add the exercise. Follow this advice, and you are more likely to reach your skinny gut goals.

Of my Skinny Gut Diet participants, Alexandra and Danielle were both avid exercisers before the diet. They were in the gym up to five times each week, but to no avail—they still struggled with weight despite their hard work. Does this story remind you of your own experience? One thing is for sure: you can't exercise your way out of a poor diet. And you can't exercise your way out of what you think is a good diet, but really isn't. Exercise is very much a part of my own life, but it's only one piece of the puzzle. Without the right diet, it's not the effective tool that it's made out to be.

Once Alexandra and Danielle began the Skinny Gut Diet, their results in the gym finally paid off. They continued to exercise, since it was already part of their routines, and they started to see the weight fall away to reveal lean muscle and skinny guts. The Skinny Gut Diet will help you finally understand food in a way that helps you achieve the body you have been working so hard for.

STRESS MANAGEMENT

If you are like me—and pretty much everyone else—you are stressed out on a regular basis. Stress is simply the norm these days, and it's wreaking havoc on our health. Managing stress is not only important to your emotional well-being but also to your digestive wellness, which is your foundation of health. Because stress induces gut imbalance, inflammation, and leaky gut, stress management is an imperative component of the Skinny Gut Diet. Everyone experiences stress at least occasionally, so it is not realistic to expect that you can eliminate stress from your life. But there are ways to manage stress that will greatly reduce its effects on you.

Identify your stressors. The first step in stress management is to identify the stressors in your life. Make a list of the stressors you experience in your life. What experiences, thoughts, feelings, and behaviors in your life stress you out? Take some time to consider all the obvious and not-so-obvious stressors. After you have made your list, carry a journal around with you for about a week so that you can identify those stressors you might not have thought to add to the list. By the end of the week, you will have a good idea of what your main stressors are.

Reduce those stressors. From your list, identify those stressors you can eliminate or reduce. That monthly lunch you schedule with an old friend who does nothing but complain the whole time? Schedule it every other month instead of monthly. The way you always respond to your mother-in-law when she criticizes your way of cooking? Let that one go. It's not likely to change, and it's not worth stressing over. Your late-night snacking habit that feels good in the moment, but that you regret afterward? Recognize that it's a behavior that ultimately stresses you out, and that you have the ability to change it. The least favorite item on your to-do list? Figure out a way to cross it off for good. Time management is crucial to helping reduce your stress level. There are only so many hours in the day. Be sure that not every minute is filled with a task.

Acknowledge unhealthy methods of coping with stress. We all have ways of dealing with stress, but some are healthier than others. If you tend to turn to habits like smoking, drinking, overeating, excessive shopping, sleeping too much, procrastinating, or taking your stress out on others, recognize that these practices are causing more damage than good.

Learn to manage the stress you cannot change. While you will certainly be able to strip away a few stressors in your life, most likely many of your stressors cannot be changed. That's a fact of modern life. Fortunately, you can still change your response to those stressors, which can go a long way toward helping you remain calm, cool, and collected. (See Resources, page 263, for a list and descriptions of effective methods of stress management that you can incorporate into your life.)

CHAPTER 14 SUMMARY

The rescue kit will help you integrate the Skinny Gut Diet anywhere, anyhow, so that you stay on track toward your weight-loss goal.

Snack Survival Guide
> ➤ Snacks are an important part of the Skinny Gut Diet because they help you get your protein throughout the day to control cravings.

Dining Out with Ease
> ➤ Dining out is not the carb trap you thought it was. There will always be options for you to choose from; you simply need to know what to look for and when to be creative.

Grocery Shopping Strategy Guide
➤ You will find that you naturally shop the perimeter when eating on the Skinny Gut Diet.

Exercise
➤ If you already have an exercise regimen in place before starting the Skinny Gut Diet, great—keep doing what you're doing. But if you are not exercising regularly at the onset of this diet, wait until you get acclimated before adding any exercise.

Stress Management
➤ Managing stress is important not only to your emotional well-being but also to your digestive wellness, which is your foundation of health.

ACKNOWLEDGMENTS

It is truly gratifying to have such an amazing team help me to create this book. The people who contribute, and the sharing of ideas, are what make a project like this one whole, fun, and successful. There are three women who were especially valuable in the development and completion of this book: Jamey Jones, Jemma Sinclaire, and Brenda Valen. They gave their support in different ways and, using their unique talents, they brought this book to completion.

Jamey Jones, you are the backbone of this book. You took my vision and direction and put it into readable form with your writing. You are gifted in so many ways, and I appreciate and love working with you. You are a bright, intelligent light who continues to work passionately on each project to bring it to fruition.

Jemma Sinclaire ran the project with all of our participants in the weight-loss program, and much more. What an organized, inspirational teacher she is. Jemma is a wonderful soul with a kind heart and a brain to go with it.

Brenda Valen is my assistant who most times knows me better than I know myself. She protects me and guides me, but most of all she is one of the most dependable people in my life. I love her like a sister and could not think of any project I do that she does not directly affect.

Dr. Leonard Smith, my friend and mentor, gives invaluable contributions to every book we write. I know I can count on Dr. Smith to make sure our message is accurate and scientifically sound. He started as a vascular surgeon and has spent the last thirty years in functional medicine. It has been truly rewarding to work with him all these years and I value his contribution to this work.

Bonnie Solow, my agent, recognized the value of this project in its infancy and encouraged me to continue developing the program. Bonnie is an inspiration to me. I love strong women, and she is definitely in that category. Bonnie, I appreciate your guidance and your support of this book.

Dominick Anfuso at Crown Publishing, thank you for believing in this manuscript. I love being able to work with you again. And to the team at Crown, all I can say is, "Wow!" What a machine in the art of selling books.

I want to thank each of the ten Skinny Gut Diet participants we worked with over the months: Alexandra, Charlie, Cynthia, Danielle, Dave, Sandi, Eva, Shirley, Teresa, and Polly. I know you thought I was the teacher, but the opposite was true. You taught me so much over the months, and you kept me inspired. Each one of you touched my heart in many ways. Working together as a group, we were able to help each other over the hurdles that come with losing weight. Each and every one of you will pass the torch, as you have seen the miracles that happen when you change your health.

Thank you to the team at ReNew Life and Advanced Naturals. You are the family who stands behind each project with me, cheering me on. Special thanks goes to the marketing team for helping us in the development of the book whenever you were called upon. We have the mutual goal of educating people to live healthier lives through better digestion, and with each book we reach more people and change more lives.

Thanks to Jim Bayne for his illustrations and graphics to help people to visualize my message, which is an important part of learning. Thank you for your creative input.

As always, thank you to my family who support me in all my

endeavors. Special thanks to Sandee, my sister, for being an early participant in the weight-loss program, as well as for being a cheerleader for the others.

Without each and every one of these wonderful people, this book could not have been written. Together, our goal is to teach and help anyone who wants to take the challenge of losing weight and changing their lives for the better by discovering their inner weight-loss secret.

APPENDIX

GUT SCIENCE WITH DR. LEONARD SMITH

Gut Bacterial Balance + Healthy Diet = Lean Individual

The link between gut microbial composition and obesity is one of the most fascinating health issues currently being studied. Jeffrey Gordon's lab, at the University of Washington, St. Louis, has consistently produced cutting-edge research that is taking our understanding of the integral role of gut balance—and its interaction with diet—on the development of obesity to fascinating places.

In another groundbreaking study led by Vanessa Ridaura, a graduate student in Gordon's lab, the team found that, "transmissible and modifiable interactions between diet and microbiota influence host biology."[1] They began by transplanting stool from four pairs of female human twins—one twin was lean and one obese in each pair—into germ-free mice. The mice were fed a standard mouse chow diet low in fat and high in fiber. The mice who received stool—and thus, the gut microbes—from the obese women accumulated more fat than did the mice who received microbes from the lean women, even though they were eating the exact same low-fat, high-fiber diet.

The mice receiving the obese microbes also exhibited higher expression of microbial genes involved in detoxification and stress response (likely because their bodies were under stress and needed

more detoxification) and increases in essential amino acids (which
the researchers later found were associated with mild glucose intolerance, perhaps the early stages of insulin resistance development, they
suggested). The mice receiving the lean microbiome exhibited higher
expression of genes involved in digestion of fibers and fermentation
to the short-chain fatty acids butyrate and propionate (due to an increase in the ability of these microbes to break down dietary fibers, a
function that has been found previously to be linked with a decrease
in body weight and fat accumulation).[2]

The researchers then repeated these studies using a culture collection, rather than the intact stool sample, from the donor human
twins. This was done to test the ability of only the culturable microbes found in stool to exhibit the same effects as the entire microbiome. As a matter of practicality, direct fecal transplantation in
humans is much more complicated than transplant of a culturable
sample that could be replicated and stored in a lab. This would eliminate the need for a human donor for each transplant, a practice that
greatly inhibits the progress not only of studies but also of the ability
for this research to make its way into the real world for use by patients
in need of a treatment for obesity. Like the mice receiving intact stool
transplants, the mice receiving the cultured collections from obese
humans accumulated more fat than those mice receiving culture collections from lean humans.

Next, the researchers placed mice who had received a culture collection from an obese woman with mice who had received a culture
collection from a lean woman. Mice are coprophagic, which is a fancy
way of saying that they eat one another's feces. Not an appetizing
thought, to be sure, but it's a fact of nature. What is important about
this is that when the "obese" mice were placed with the "lean" mice
and fed the same low-fat, high-fiber chow, the obese mice began to
inherit the microbes from the lean mice and lost the fat they had
accumulated, becoming more like the "lean" mice. Very interestingly,
the "lean" mice did not inherit the gut microbes of the "obese" mice,
nor did they gain any fat. The microbes they had inherited from the

lean human protected them against invasion of microbes from the "obese" mice, which protected them against accumulating fat.

The "lean" mice were found to have higher levels of *Bacteroides*, not surprisingly, given what you have already learned. The researchers tracked the invasion of certain members of *Bacteroides* from the "lean" to the "obese" mice while they were cohoused, suggesting that these bacteria may be responsible for the protection against obesity. The researchers hypothesized that *Bacteroides* (a subgroup of Bacteroidetes) were efficient invaders of "obese" microbiotas because they were able to occupy unoccupied niches in the intestines of the "obese" mice, which did not have as rich a microbial diversity as the "lean" mice.

Next the researchers replicated the cohousing studies and fed the mice a diet made with foods that replicate a low-fat, high-fruit, and high-vegetable intake, characteristic of a "healthy" diet. The mice that received culture collections from the obese women had increased body mass and fat accumulation even on the "healthy" diet as compared to those mice that received culture collections from lean women, just as they did when eating the regular mouse chow. Also similarly, when cohoused, the "lean" mice were protected against obesity, and when the "obese" mice ingested bacteria from the lean mice, they again reverted to a lean profile.

Finally, the researchers again repeated the study, only this time they fed the mice a diet high in saturated fat and low in fruits and vegetables—more reminiscent of the Standard American Diet (SAD). The mice receiving culture collections from obese humans still gained more fat and body mass compared to those receiving culture collections from lean humans while eating this diet. When they were cohoused, however, something different happened. The "obese" mice were no longer able to receive the bacteria from the "lean" mice, and did not revert back to being lean. The SAD diet completely relinquished the ability of the "obese" mice to receive beneficial bacteria from the "lean" mice and revert back to being lean.

Let me rephrase that because it's an important point: Eating a Standard American Diet prevented the "obese" mice from being colonized with beneficial bacteria from the lean mice, and also prevented them from losing weight. Here's the bottom line: *Not only do you need to balance your gut by taking probiotics and fiber, but you also need to support that balance with the right diet.*

A diet high in nonstarchy vegetables and low-sugar fruits, healthy fats, proteins, nuts, and seeds will feed the beneficial bacteria in your gut that protect you against disease, including obesity. Adding probiotics and prebiotic fibers to this diet will help ensure you house the right microbes in your gut.

Ecosystems Are Complex

While I wish that I could tell you that all you have to do is boost your Bacteroidetes bacteria and lower your Firmicutes, it's not quite that simple. There is more going on in your gut than a simple division into two groups of bacteria. You have already learned that the Bacteroidetes and Firmicutes are large groups of bacteria called phyla. All living organisms are classified according to groups, beginning with the largest groups: kingdoms. Remember high school biology—the animal kingdom, bacteria kingdom, plant kingdom? Each kingdom is further separated into groups called phyla (phylum, singular). Under the bacteria kingdom are a number of phyla. When it comes to the bacteria that live inside of us, the main phyla identified thus far are Firmicutes, Bacteroidetes, Actinobacteria, and Proteobacteria. The following table lists the top four human bacterial phyla along with the representative genera (genus, singular).

Phylum/Phyla	Genus/Genera
Firmicutes	Ruminococcus
	Clostridium
	Streptococcus
	Enterococcus
	Lactobacillus

Phylum/Phyla	Genus/Genera
Bacteroidetes	Bacteroides
	Prevotella
Actinobacteria	Bifidobacterium
Proteobacteria	Desulfovibrio
	Escherichia
	Helicobacter

As you can see from the above table, genera are groups of bacteria (only some of which are represented here). Most of the effects of your gut microbes occur at the level of these smaller groups. You have already learned about *Lactobacillus* and *Bifidobacterium,* two of the most beneficial bacteria in the human gut. You may have also noticed that *Lactobacillus* is actually under the Firmicutes phyla and *Bifidobacterium* is not in either the Firmicutes or Bacteroidetes phyla but, rather, in an entirely different phylum called Actinobacteria. As I said, your inner ecosystem is more complicated than a simple division into two groups of bacteria. While the overall Firmicutes-to-Bacteroidetes ratio is important, we must also look at the individual genus groups to fully understand gut balance. Again, Bifidobacteria are not in the Bacteroidetes phylum, and Lactobacilli are in the Firmicutes phylum, and yet their importance to our health and to the protection against obesity, as well as many other health conditions, has been well demonstrated. So, generally speaking, shifting your overall bacteria toward the "lean gut type"—more Bacteroidetes and fewer Firmicutes—along with replenishing your gut with Bifidobacteria and Lactobacilli will be the best approach for achieving gut balance.

Gut Bacterial Diversity and Metabolism

There are more factors that contribute to the development of obesity and related conditions than simply what we eat and how much energy we expend. The very notion of calories in, calories out is not what it seems—at least, not at face value. As researchers are discovering, your gut microbes have more to do with your metabolism than you might ever have imagined. A study published in the journal *Nature* gives us a closer look at how our gut inhabitants affect our propensity to develop obesity and related conditions.[3]

The researchers looked at the gut microbial composition, including the number of microbial genes, of 292 obese and non-obese Danish individuals. They were able to separate the individuals into two groups based on their number of microbial genes—what they called *bacterial richness*. Those with the highest gene count had the highest bacterial richness, and vice versa. They found that those with the lowest bacterial richness (23 percent of the individuals) also had more abdominal fat, insulin resistance, high insulin, increased triglycerides, decreased HDL-cholesterol ("good" cholesterol), and increased C-reactive protein (hsCRP—a marker of inflammation) when compared to the group with high bacterial richness. What this means is that those people with the lowest diversity of gut microbes were more likely to have elevated levels of a range of biomarkers normally found in people with obesity, diabetes, heart disease, and other inflammatory chronic diseases. This suggests that the gut microbes may be responsible for the metabolic imbalances.

Gut balance is determined not only by the right amounts of good and bad bacteria but also by the diversity of bacteria. After all, the more diverse our gut microbes, the more resilient they will be under stressful conditions. Bacterial richness is a reflection of bacterial diversity and, thus, represents gut balance.

In the people with low bacterial richness, the researchers found 46 different bacteria groups (genera) to be more abundant; these include such potential pathogens as *Campylobacter, Porphyromonas, Ruminococcus,* and *Staphylococcus.* In the people with high bacterial richness, they found an abundance of *Faecalibacterium, Bifidobacterium, Lactobacillus, Methanobrevibacter,* and more. You may notice two stars in that last group—*Lactobacillus* and *Bifidobacterium.* Because of the wide range of human health benefits of these probiotics, it is no surprise that they were found to be abundant in healthy people who had higher bacterial richness.

The researchers also found that those who had low bacterial richness exhibited the potential to produce metabolites with possible deleterious health effects, including the ability to produce carcinogens—yes, your gut bacteria can produce carcinogens, especially when your gut is out of balance. On the other hand, those people who had high bacterial richness exhibited the potential to produce organic acids known to be beneficial to health, including the short-chain fatty acids lactate, propionate, acetate, and butyrate.

Those with low bacterial richness (shall we call them bacterially poor?) showed the following characteristics:

- Reduction in the butyrate-producing bacteria (butyrate nourishes the cells of the intestinal lining)
- Increased potential for mucous degradation (the mucous lining protects the intestinal lining from damage)
- Reduced hydrogen and methane production potential combined with increased hydrogen sulfide formation potential (hydrogen sulfide is a toxic gas produced by pathogenic bacteria)
- Increase abundance of Campylobacter/Shigella (both potential pathogens)
- Increased potential for oxidative stress (production of peroxidase)

About these characteristics the researchers stated:

Overall, this suggests that [those individuals with low bacterial richness] harbor an inflammation-associated microbiota. Together, these analyses suggest that the [low bacterial richness] individuals are featured by metabolic disturbances known to put them at increased risk of pre-diabetes, type 2 diabetes, and ischemic cardiovascular disorders. We propose that an imbalance of potentially pro- and anti-inflammatory bacterial species triggers low-grade inflammation and insulin resistance.[4]

Low bacterial richness has also been found in patients with inflammatory bowel disease, elderly patients with inflammation, and obese individuals. In animal studies, this reduced bacterial richness has been induced by repeated antibiotic use. In humans, antibiotic use during childhood has been found to lead to increased risk of later being overweight, possibly due to a reduction in bacterial richness.[5] In the Danish study, *the obese individuals with low bacterial richness gained more weight than did the individuals with high bacterial richness.*

As the authors of the Danish study state, "Obesity is not just obesity." There is more to the story. Even lean people can harbor the wrong microbes, or have a low diversity of microbes, and be more at risk for chronic health conditions normally associated with obesity. This study will certainly lead to more investigation into the diversity of our gut microbes, and more specifically, how those microbes interact to produce health or disease.

Metabolic Endotoxemia

You have already learned that bacterial toxins are produced inside the gut. One particular digestive toxin, an endotoxin known as lipopolysaccharide (LPS), has been found to induce inflammation that leads to obesity.[6] LPS is mostly produced by Gram-negative bacteria in the gut. Increased levels of LPS endotoxin in the bloodstream (due to gut imbalance coupled with a poor diet) is known as *metabolic endotoxemia*, a condition that has been found to induce many of the features of obesity. Metabolic endotoxemia directly triggers inflammation, beginning with the lining of blood vessels and continuing with a downstream effect of increasing blood sugar levels, insulin resistance, and fat accumulation, all associated with metabolic syndrome and obesity. The result is weight gain. Lowering LPS levels has been suggested as a potent strategy for the control of metabolic diseases, particularly obesity and diabetes.[7] How do you lower LPS levels to reverse all of this damage? You balance your gut by increasing the good bacteria. You see, your gut microbes control the permeability, or leakiness, of your intestinal lining. Good bacteria protect the lining from invaders and bad bacteria damage the lining, promote inflammation, and increase the leakiness of the gut.

> **High-fat, high-sugar diet ⇢ Change in gut microbes ⇢**
> **Leaky gut ⇢ Endotoxins absorbed ⇢ Metabolic endotoxemia**
> **⇢ Silent inflammation ⇢ OBESITY**

Metabolic endotoxemia (excess LPS endotoxins in the blood) is caused by gut imbalance and is accompanied by leaky gut, blood sugar abnormalities, weight gain, fat accumulation, and inflammation.[8] Metabolic endotoxemia's perfect storm of gut imbalance, inflammation, and leaky gut is at the heart of the obesity epidemic, with leaky gut acting as the doorway to destruction. In fact, metabolic endotoxemia has been linked to increased insulin and triglyceride levels as well as lower HDL ("good") cholesterol levels in patients with obesity and type 2 diabetes. Even in healthy people, leaky gut has been linked to the accumulation of abdominal fat.[9] Abdominal fat, also called visceral fat, is strongly related to inflammation, insulin resistance, and the development of obesity and related chronic diseases. Many vicious cycles exist, each feeding into the other, and spiraling toward chronic disease. To truly make a dent in the problem, we must first address the underlying gut imbalance.

In another interesting study linking gut bacteria to obesity-related conditions, over 3,200 people were followed for nine years.[10] Those individuals with the highest levels of bacteria genes detected in the bloodstream (which is an indication that increased amounts of bacteria "leaked" though the intestinal lining) were more likely to develop diabetes and accumulate abdominal fat when compared to those with the lowest levels. Further, the detected bacteria genes of those who developed diabetes were mostly composed of proteobacteria, a group of bacteria represented by many pathogens that produce endotoxins. This is another indication that gut imbalance increases endotoxins and leads to leaky gut, which can lead to obesity. It's as though once the gut bacteria become imbalanced, a chain of events occurs that destroys digestive health and sets you up for weight gain. To reverse this trend, you must start at the very beginning by rebalancing the gut.

Taking these studies one step further, researchers from the Netherlands actually transplanted intestinal microbes from lean people into the digestive tracts of male recipients with metabolic syndrome (metabolic syndrome is the precursor to diabetes).[11] Six weeks after receiving these microbes, insulin sensitivity increased (which indicates an improvement of the metabolic syndrome) along with the amount of butyrate-producing bacteria in their intestines when compared to men who had received a transplant of their own microbes. Remember that butyrate is the short-chain fatty acid that nourishes the intestinal lining. It is produced by Bifidobacteria, among other beneficial bacteria. Interesting to note, butyrate has been found to have an appetite-suppressing effect, also beneficial for people who want to lose weight.[12] This is a pivotal study in the investigation of the human gut microbiota. It shows the amazing response to altering gut microbes for the better, and it helps confirm in humans what has been found in so many animal models. Now we know that our own microbes behave in much the same way as they do in these animal studies. Further, it helps prove that balancing gut bacteria positively affects metabolic health. Insulin sensitivity of our body's cells is crucial for optimal health and prevention of diseases associated with high blood sugar, including obesity, type 2 diabetes, and even Alzheimer's disease (which has been dubbed type 3 diabetes).

Further research with regard to the short-chain fatty acids (butyrate being one), shows that healthy levels of acetate and propionate in the stool and blood will bind to the cell surface receptors GPR43 and GPR41 on colon epithelial cells and various white blood cells. This connection profoundly modulates the immune response. In fact, animals with low levels of acetate and propionate or low GPR43 receptor number or function are not likely to survive serious microbial threats (infections) and at the same time will overreact to normal food and bacterial antigens, thereby creating allergies and/ or asthma.[13] On the other hand, butyrate can also bind to GPR41, as well as be taken up into colonic and immune cells. In the colon cells, butyrate goes to the cell nucleus, attaches to the epigenome, and blocks histone deacetylase, which inhibits NF-kappaB and thereby decreases inflammation and promotes apoptosis (death) of precancerous colon cells.[14] The implication here is huge. Consuming adequate amounts of fiber and having enough beneficial bacteria in the gut results in far less Crohn's disease, ulcerative colitis, and colon polyps and/or cancer of the colon. Thus, we can see that research is continuing to show that the natural order of a high-fiber diet is needed for health and survival.

As we continue to look at the natural order of life, it will reveal many clues about how critical different parts are to overall function. From the perspective of a senior, perhaps one of the major reasons people over 70 have troubles with their intestinal tract (and much more) has to do with the sun. It is known that the ability for those over 70 to make vitamin D decreases by about 70 percent. Animal models have shown that a marked decrease in vitamin D and vitamin D receptors in the intestinal epithelium will lower the trans-epithelial electrical resistance and also lead to disruptions of epithelial junctions, both of which lead to leaky gut.[15] The lack of vitamin D also literally will cause changes in the gut microbiota, which can lead to dysbiosis. Furthermore, even if commensal bacteria leak through the intestinal lining, it will cause major immune disturbances leading to the various systematic diseases we have discussed in the book. I predict that further study of vitamin D and vitamin D receptors in the gut will lead to much better understanding for prevention and management of all types of inflammation of the intestinal tract.[16]

In conclusion, I must remind everyone that most of our microbiome is still unculturable. Even what is culturable from the feces may not accurately represent what is going on in the metabolically active healthy colon. There is still much to understand with regard to the content and functionality of our microbiome. Columbus took the *Santa Maria* to discover the New World—today we take a jet.

I would guess we are still at the Columbus stage in our full understanding of the microbiome.

FAQS

How much weight can I expect to lose?

How much weight you lose depends on a number of factors. In general, the more weight you have to lose, the faster you will lose the weight. You can expect to lose *at least* 1 to 2 pounds each week on the Skinny Gut Diet. The first two weeks, it is common for people to lose more than that.

Do I have to eat only products that are labeled "gluten-free"?

If you have a gluten sensitivity, you will want to avoid gluten by purchasing products that are gluten-free. Many people with gluten sensitivity do not realize they have it. If you find that by removing gluten from your diet you feel better (and when you reintroduce gluten you notice digestive or other symptoms), then you should steer clear of gluten. If you would like to be tested for gluten sensitivity, see Resources, page 257, for a test that I recommend.

Do I have to take the supplements?

The Skinny Gut supplements are an important part of the Skinny Gut Diet. The H.O.P.E. Formula will help to balance your gut in conjunction with the diet. They work hand in hand. If you do not take the supplements, you will not experience the full benefits of the Skinny Gut Diet.

What if I can't stand fermented foods?

For some people, fermented foods are an acquired taste. The flavor of these foods is different from that of any other foods. Fortunately, after you begin to incorporate fermented foods into your diet, you will find that you grow to enjoy the taste. Stick with it, and your experience will change.

I'm constipated. What am I doing wrong?

You may not be eating enough fiber. You want to get *at least* 35 grams of fiber every day from your diet and supplements. That won't be a problem if you are eating five to nine servings of nonstarchy vegetables and low-sugar fruits every day (you might want to get closer to nine than five if you are constipated) and taking your fiber supplement. In some cases, dietary changes can create a sluggish bowel in the beginning. An herbal laxative may be needed in this case. In addition, probiotics and fermented foods play an important role. They improve your bacterial balance and help restore regularity. If you do not experience a daily bowel movement, you are constipated and you will not achieve weight loss as easily as you would if you did have regular bowel movements. It is critical that you properly address constipation.

All this fiber makes me gassy. What should I do?

At first, you can introduce fiber gradually. Start by eating five servings of nonstarchy vegetables and low-sugar fruits each day and work your way up as time goes on and your digestive system adjusts. Likewise, start by taking one serving of fiber per day and increasing it as you adjust. In addition, taking a digestive enzyme with every meal—and snacks if you are feeling gassy or as though you aren't digesting well—will help to break down fibrous foods so that you don't get gassy.

RESOURCES

Foods

Fermented Foods
Beagle Bay Organics sauerkraut
　　and kimchi
Chobani plain Greek yogurt
Lifeway kefir

Crackers (in moderation)
Mary's Gone Crackers
Go Raw Flax Snax
Crunchmaster Multiseed Crackers

Sweeteners and Sweets
Monk Fruit in the Raw
Sweet Drops stevia
ChocoPerfection chocolate bars

Pasta Substitutes
Explore Asian mung bean, black bean, and soybean low-carb
　　pastas
Nasoya shirataki low-carb pasta

Almond Flour
Honeyville almond flour

Coconut Butter/Manna
Nutiva, Artisana

Tools

Vegetable spiralizer
Sundesa blender bottle (shaker cup)
Slow cooker

Blenders
   Hamilton Beach single-serve blender
   Ninja Kitchen System Pulse
   Vitamix
   Blendtec
   Magic Bullet
Igloo Playmate Gripper Lunchbox
Pyrex 1-cup storage round
Pyrex 4-cup rectangle container
Taylor Digital Kitchen Scale

Online Resources

Elana's Pantry (ElanasPantry.com): Grain-free cooking and
   baking. Where honey and agave are used, you can substitute
   lo han or stevia using a simple conversion. Her Pecan
   Shortbread Cookies are great to keep on hand. Store the
   dough in the freezer for a ready-to-bake treat anytime.
Probiotic Research (Probiotic-Research.com): Library of original
   abstracts of published, peer-reviewed, human probiotic
   research.

Nutrition Data

Self-Nutrition Data
Database of nutrition information for most common foods
NutritionData.Self.com

Nutrition Data Book
The Complete Book of Food Counts by Corinne Netzer

Supplements

H.O.P.E. Formula from ReNew Life Formulas
ReNewLife.com

UltimateFlora.com

NorwegianGoldFishOils.com

FiberSmart.com

DigestSmart.com

Organic Acacia Fiber (Organic Clear Fiber)

Organic Acacia Fiber with Fruit

Non-GMO Corn Fiber (Clear Fiber)

Super Critical Omega

Ultimate Flora Probiotics

DigestSmart Critical Care digestive enzymes

Ultimate Shake

Two-week cleanse: First Cleanse

Thirty-day cleanse: Cleanse Smart

Cleanse More

IntestiNew (L-glutamine)

Sweet Life lo han (monk fruit) sweetener

Doctor's Best Nutritional Supplements

Metagenics (Metagenics.com)

Pure Encapsulations (PureEncapsulations.com)

Standard Process (StandardProcess.com)

Life Flo (Life-Flo.com)

Books

By Brenda Watson, C.N.C., and Leonard Smith, M.D.
Heart of Perfect Health
The Road to Perfect Health
The Fiber35 Diet
The Detox Strategy
Gut Solutions
Renew Your Life
Essential Cleansing
The H.O.P.E. Formula

- Choose organic meats to avoid the hormones and antibiotics found in nonorganic meats.
- Choose unprocessed foods to avoid preservatives, dyes, nitrates, and nitrites.
- Choose natural products to clean your home environment. There are many brands on the market that work very well and do not contain harsh chemicals. Also, remember to choose skin and hair products that contain minimal chemicals and dyes.
- Change the air-conditioning filters in your home often. Get the ducts cleaned annually. Use plants such as spider, aloe, and philodendrons to help filter your household air.
- Install a total-home water filter to help eliminate the chlorine and other chemicals found in your water.

Step 2: Remove Toxins from Your Body

Getting rid of the toxins already in your ͅ   little more difficult. I have already told you that the b   ͅoxins in fat cells. The question is: What can we do   ͅns out of the fat cells and out of the body? The ͅ   ͅfication and cleansing, which you can do throug'   ͅtions that we'll explore shortly.

Detoxific   ͅng are crucial to good health. In addition t   ͅins, the very act of living creates poisons t'   ͅed out of the body. Detoxification and cleans-ii   ͅterms for the collection and elimination of these poi.

Saun . Saunas, as well as steam baths and hot bathtub soaks, are great for sweating out unwanted toxins. Sweating occurs naturally during physical activity, but it can also be induced through either a sauna or a bath. The health benefits of saunas in particular are numerous. The skin is the largest organ of your body and a prime participant in elimination. Because of its size and area, it actually eliminates more cellular waste—through the pores—than the colon and kidneys combined.

Green Drinks. Green vegetable juices are an excellent way to cleanse. Short-term cleansing, such as a one-day green drink cleanse can be a great way to give your body a digestive rest along with a nutrient boost. Incorporating juices into your daily routine is a great way to get a high concentration of nutrients from vegetables. See the green drinks recipes, pages 144 to 145, in Chapter 10.

Herbal Cleansing and Detoxification. I have always been a big fan of using herbs, supplements, and diet to improve the efficiency of the detoxification process. I have seen great successes in my clinics with people who have lost weight and improved their health. Based on your level of toxicity I would suggest a program of herbs, supplements, and food that can help you maximize your weight loss by improving each of the seven channels of detoxification: colon, liver, lungs, lymph, kidneys, skin, and blood.

Most cleansing and detoxification kits contain two formulas in a single box. The first bottle usually is a detoxification formula containing natural herbs that help pull toxins from the organs. The second bottle contains different herbs and minerals that help the colon eliminate the toxins more efficiently. You will also want to add extra fiber to your diet during cleansing because fiber helps absorb and sweep toxins out of the colon. There are many approaches to cleansing and detoxification. Depending on your individual needs and preferences, you will want to choose a two-week or thirty-day cleanse as described below:

Two-Week Cleanse. If you are a first-time cleanser, or if you have not cleansed in the last six months, or if you have daily bowel movements, you'll want to select a whole-herb cleanse that gently supports all the channels of elimination. This support is best provided with a two-part formula: (1) an evening formula to encourage mild elimination through the bowel using a variety of herbs (like marshmallow root, rhubarb root, and buckthorn bark); and (2) a morning formula that contains a synergistic blend of a variety of herbs (mostly liver-supporting) to support the remaining organs of elimination. (See Resources, page 256, for my recommended products.)

Thirty-Day Cleanse. If you have completed an internal cleanse before or simply want a longer cleanse, or if you are constipated, your best choice is a thirty-day, total-body cleanse that contains high-potency herbal extracts and whole herbs designed to support the body's seven channels of elimination. Here again, you'll want to look for a two-part formula: (1) an evening formula that contains herbs and magnesium hydroxide to hydrate and enhance elimination through the bowel, and (2) a morning formula that blends a variety of whole herbs with high-potency powdered extracts to support the remaining channels of elimination. (See Resources, page 256, for my recommended products.)

Colon Hydrotherapy. As a colon therapist, I practiced colonics for over fifteen years. A colonic is basically an extended and more complete form of an enema. Colon hydrotherapy involves repeated infusions of filtered, warm water into all segments of the colon by a certified colon therapist. Colon hydrotherapists are trained to use massage techniques to help relax the abdominal muscles and ensure that all areas of the colon are adequately irrigated and cleansed. Therapeutic benefits of colon hydrotherapy include improved tone of colonic muscles, reduced stagnation of intestinal contents, and reduced toxic waste absorption. Always look for a colon hydrotherapist who has been certified by the International Association of Colon Hydrotherapy (I-ACT), and make sure that the therapist uses FDA-approved equipment with disposable nozzles and filtered water.

Acid Blocker Recovery

Long-term use of acid-blocking medications is associated with increased infections such as *Clostridium difficile* (*C. diff*), pneumonia, *H. pylori*, and Candida overgrowth. Sudden discontinued use of these medications can have a rebound effect, however, involving overproduction of stomach acid. Therefore, gradual weaning off the medication is best. The following protocol will help you to regain control of your digestive symptoms so that you can manage your health naturally without the harmful effects of long-term blockage of stomach acid production. Let your health-care physician know that you are concerned about the harmful effects of long-term acid blocking medications and that you are looking for a safer, more natural solution to your health problem.

It takes seven days for the effects of acid-blocking medications to diminish in the body. For this reason, it is best to lower the dosage of the medication before discontinuing use.

First seven days: Take acid-blocking medication at half the normal dose. In addition, take the following supplements:

- 5,000–10,000 mg L-glutamine powder along with 200 billion cultures of probiotics daily on an empty stomach first thing in the morning
- High-potency digestive enzymes containing at least 100,000 H.U.T. protease with every meal and large snacks
- If heartburn is experienced initially, use a natural heartburn formula temporarily.

Most people who have been on long-term acid blockers will have hypochlorhydria (low stomach acid). If you do not experience any heartburn while following these suggestions, begin taking a digestive enzyme that includes HCl (hydrochloric acid) with meals after you finish the first round of digestive enzymes. Hydrochloric acid is necessary in the stomach for the absorption of key nutrients.

A small percentage of people will have hyperchlorhydria (high stomach acid), often due to stress and excess caffeine consumption. It is best to properly manage stress (see Stress Management Techniques below) and reduce or eliminate caffeine intake before beginning the acid blocker recovery.

If you experience uncomfortable symptoms while following this protocol, discontinue the process and consult your doctor. After seven days, you can either reduce your dosage by half again or you can try to stop the medication entirely. Continue to take the supplements on a daily basis to support the health of your upper and lower digestive tracts.

Stress Management Techniques

Healthy diet. Adopt a healthy diet as a way to maintain optimal total-body health. What you eat affects your health and mood, so choose the healthiest foods to put into your body so that you have the proper fuel to get you through your day. I designed the Skinny Gut Diet to support your mental well-being as much as your overall well-being because I recognize it as a crucial step to a vital, healthy life.

Exercise. Get moving as a way to relieve stress. Find a physical activity you enjoy and try to incorporate it into your life at least five days each week. Exercise releases endorphins, the body's euphoric neurotransmitters, and helps to balance the stress response. Yoga, tai chi, and qi gong are particularly beneficial stress-relieving forms of exercise because they address physical, mental, and emotional fitness.

Go outside. The healing power of nature is a potent stress reliever. Connecting to nature simply by gardening in your yard, walking through the park, sitting near a lake, or spending time at the beach is not only good for stress reduction but also for your physical health. Take time on a regular basis to go outside and take in the beauty you encounter. Better yet, take your exercise routine outside and you'll not only get a great workout, but you'll do it in an environment that can boost your mood.

Support. A good support system goes a long way toward helping relieve stress. Having someone to talk to is one of the most important ways to relieve stress. Support could come from family, friends, a counselor, support groups, or a spiritual or religious center. Build your support system so it's there when you need it.

Sleep. Lack of sleep is often the result of stress, and it also brings on stress, creating yet another vicious cycle that leads to poor health. Most people need at least seven to eight hours of sleep so that the body can function optimally. To help you sleep better, try to go to bed and wake up around the same time each day, don't drink caffeine or eat a big meal right before bed, and don't work while in bed. These sleep hygiene practices can help you get a good night sleep on a regular basis.

Hobbies. If you have a hobby that you really enjoy, make time for it as a way to reduce stress. Cooking, dancing, singing in a chorus, photography—the list of hobbies is endless. Is there something you have always wanted to learn, but didn't? Consider a new hobby as a way to blow off steam. If you find better stress relief by *doing* rather than by being still, a hobby may be the perfect activity for you.

Mindfulness skills training. Mindfulness training helps to bring about our awareness of, and attention to, the present moment. By being aware of what happens on a moment-to-moment basis, you can improve your physical and emotional well-being. Mindfulness can be cultivated through mindful sitting meditation, mindful walking, mindful eating, and mindful doing-whatever-it-is-that-you're-doing. One specific program, mindfulness-based stress reduction (MBSR) developed by Jon Kabat-Zinn, teaches mindfulness skills in a variety of formats and may be helpful.

Cognitive behavioral therapy (CBT). The psychotherapeutic approach utilizes goal-oriented systematic, present-moment-based methods to address a variety of disorders. The CBT strategies help to change thought patterns as a way to reduce stress.

Relaxation methods. There are many different relaxation methods, all of which can help relieve stress. Deep breathing, progressive muscle relaxation, meditation, biofeedback, massage, guided imagery, and aromatherapy are a few relaxation methods that may be helpful.

Acupuncture, acupressure, and Reiki. Stress may be the result of energetic imbalances in the body that can be corrected with acupuncture, a traditional Chinese medical procedure using small needles lightly placed into certain points on the body; acupressure, similar to acupuncture except that pressure is used instead of needles; and Reiki, a Japanese traditional healing method that involves using the hands as a way to manipulate the energy of the body. Each of these methods stimulates the flow of energy, correcting imbalances. Both emotional and physical manifestations of stress can be treated with these methods, usually over several treatment sessions.

Emotional freedom technique (EFT). During an EFT session, the individual focuses on a particular concern while tapping on meridian points of the body. A wide range of well-respected integrative health practitioners and doctors have had effective results with this technique and recommend it widely.

NOTES

Chapter 1: A Remarkable Discovery—Guess Who's Coming to Dinner?

1. A. M. O'Hara and F. Shanahan, "The Gut Flora As a Forgotten Organ," *European Molecular Biology Organization Reports* 7, no. 7 (July 2006) : 688–93.
2. G. Taubes, *Good Calories, Bad Calories* (New York: First Anchor Books, 2008).
3. P. D. Cani, R. Bibiloni, C. Knauf, et al., "Changes in Gut Microbiota Control Metabolic Endotoxemia-Induced Inflammation in High-Fat Diet-Induced Obesity and Diabetes in Mice," *Diabetes* 57, no. 6 (June 2008): 1470–81.

Chapter 2: Gut Bacteria—The Surprising Weight-Loss Solution

1. R. E. Ley, P. J. Turnbaugh, S. Klein, et al., "Microbial Ecology: Human Gut Microbes Associated with Obesity," *Nature* 444 (December 2006): 1022–23.
2. Ibid.
3. C. De Filippo, D. Cavalieri, M. Di Paola, et al., "Impact of Diet in Shaping Gut Microbiota Revealed by a Comparative Study in Children from Europe and Rural Africa," *Proceedings of the National Academy of Sciences of the United States* 107, no. 33 (August 2010): 14691–96.
4. F. Bäckhed, H. Ding, T. Wang, et al., "The Gut Microbiota As an Environmental Factor that Regulates Fat Storage," *Proceedings of the National Academy of Sciences of the United States* 101, no. 44 (November 2004): 15718–23.
5. P. J. Turnbaugh, R. E. Ley, M.A. Mahowald, et al., "An Obesity-Associated Gut Microbiome with Increased Capacity for Energy Harvest," *Nature* 444 (December 2006): 1027–31.
6. R. E. Ley, F. Bäckhed, P. J. Turnbaugh, et al., "Obesity Alters Gut Microbial Ecology," *Proceedings of the National Academy of Sciences of the United States* 102, no. 31 (August 2005): 11070–75.
7. P. J. Turnbaugh, M. Hamady, T. Yatsuneko, et al., "A Core Gut Microbiome in Obese and Lean Twins," *Nature* 457 (January 2009): 480–84.
8. I. Nadal, A. Santacruz, A. Marcos, et al., "Shifts in Clostridia, Bacteroides and Immunoglobulin-Coating Fecal Bacteria Associated with Weight Loss in Obese Adolescents," *International Journal of Obesity* 33, no. 7 (July 2009):

758–67; C. De Filippo, et al., "Impact of Diet in Shaping Gut Microbiota," 14691–96.

9. Audrey Eyton, *The F-Plan Diet* (New York: Crown, 1982), 18.

10. E. Wisker, A. Maltz, and W. Feldheim, "Metabolizable Energy of Diets Low or High in Dietary Fiber from Cereals when Eaten by Humans," *Journal of Nutrition* 118, no. 8 (August 1988): 945–52.

11. P. D. Cani, N. M. Delzenne, J. Amar, et al., "Role of Gut Microflora in the Development of Obesity and Insulin Resistance Following High-Fat Diet Feeding," *Pathologie Biologie* 56, no. 5 (July 2008): 305–309; S. Thuy, R. Ladurner, V. Volynets, et al., "Nonalcoholic Fatty Liver Disease in Humans Is Associated with Increased Plasma Endotoxin and Plasminogen Activator Inhibitor 1 Concentrations and with Fructose Intake," *Journal of Nutrition* 138, no. 8 (August 2008): 1452–55; M. Heyman and J. F. Desjeux, "Cytokine-Induced Alteration of the Epithelial Barrier to Food Antigens in Disease," *Annals of the New York Academy of Sciences* 915 (2000): 304–11.

12. P. D. Cani, A. M. Neyrinck, F. Fava, et al., "Selective Increases of Bifidobacteria in Gut Microflora Improve High-Fat-Diet-Induced Diabetes in Mice Through a Mechanism Associated with Endotoxaemia," *Diabetologia* 50, no. 11 (November 2007): 2374–83; N. M. Delzenne, A. M. Neyrinck, F. Bäckhed, et al., "Targeting Gut Microbiota in Obesity: Effects of Prebiotics and Probiotics," *National Review of Endocrinology* 7, no. 11 (August 2011): 639–46.

13. V. Norris, F. Molina, and A. T. Gewirtz, "Hypothesis: Bacteria Control Host Appetites," *Journal of Bacteriology* 195, no. 3 (February 2013): 411–16.

14. J. M. Goodson, D. Groppo, S. Halem, et al., "Is Obesity an Oral Bacterial Disease?" *Journal of Dental Research* 88, no. 6 (June 2009): 519–23.

15. H. Zhang, J. K. DiBaise, A. Zuccolo, et al., "Human Gut Microbiota in Obesity and After Gastric Bypass," *Proceedings of the National Academy of Science of the United States* 106, no. 7 (February 2009): 2365–70.

16. A. P. Liou, M. Paziuk, J. M. Luevano Jr., et al., "Conserved Shifts in the Gut Microbiota Due to Gastric Bypass Reduce Host Weight and Adiposity," *Science Translational Medicine* 5, no. 178 (March 2013): 178ra41.

17. G. A. Woodard, B. Encarnacion, J. R. Downey, et al., "Probiotics Improve Outcomes after Roux-en-Y Gastric Bypass Surgery: A Prospective Randomized Trial," *Journal of Gastrointestinal Surgery* 13, no. 7 (July 2009): 1198–204.

Chapter 3: Where Did It All Go Wrong?

1. G. Musso, R. Gambino, and M. Cassader, et al., "Obesity, Diabetes, and Gut Microbiota: The Hygiene Hypothesis Expanded?" *Diabetes Care* 33, no. 10 (October 2010): 2277–84.

2. M. M. Gronlund, O. P. Lehtonen, E. Eerola, et al., "Fecal Microflora in Healthy Infants Born by Different Methods of Delivery: Permanent Changes in Intestinal Flora after Cesarean Delivery," *Journal of Pediatric Gastroenterology and Nutrition* 28, no. 1 (January 1999): 19–25.

3. M. Kalliomaki, "Early Differences in Fecal Microbiota Composition in Children May Predict Overweight," *American Journal of Clinical Nutrition* 87, no. 3 (March 2008): 534–38.

4. A. C. Lundell, I. Adlerberth, E. Lindberg, et al., "Increased Levels of Circulating Soluble CD14 but Not CD83 in Infants Are Associated with Early Intestinal Colonization with Staphylococcus aureus," *Clinical and Experimental Allergy* 37, no. 1 (January 2007): 62–71; P. D. Cani, J. Amar, M. A. Iglesias, et al., "Metabolic Endotoxemia Initiates Obesity and Insulin Resistance," *Diabetes* 56, no. 7 (July 2007): 1761–72.

5. M. C. Collado, E. Isolauri, K. Laitinen, et al., "Distinct Composition of Gut Microbiota During Pregnancy in Overweight and Normal-Weight Women," *American Journal of Clinical Nutrition* 88, no. 4 (October 2008): 894–99.

6. J. B. German, S. L. Freeman, C. B. Lebrilla, et al., "Human Milk Oligosaccharides: Evolution, Structures and Bioselectivity as Substrates for Intestinal Bacteria," *Nestle Nutrition Workshop Series Pediatric Program* 62 (2008): 205-18; discussion 218–22. M. Gueimonde, K. Laitinen, S. Salminen, et al., "Breast Milk: A Source of Bifidobacteria for Infant Gut Development and Maturation?" *Neonatology* 92, no. 1 (2007): 64–66.

7. K. G. Kinsella, "Changes in Life Expectancy 1900-1990, *American Journal of Clinical Nutrition* 55, no. 6 (June 1992, Suppl): 1196S–202S.

8. G. Musso, et al., "Obesity, Diabetes, and Gut Microbiota, 2277–84.

9. M. C. Noverr and G. B. Huffnagle, "The 'Microflora Hypothesis' of Allergic Diseases," *Clinical and Experimental Allergy* 35, no. 12 (December 2005): 1511–20.

10. G. Musso, et al., "Obesity, Diabetes, and Gut Microbiota."

11. L. Dethlefsen, S. Huse, M. L. Sogin, et al., "The Pervasive Effects of an Antibiotic on the Human Gut Microbiota, As Revealed by Deep 16S rRNA Sequencing," *Public Library of Science Biology* 6, no. 11 (November 2008): e280; L. Dethlefsen and D. A. Relman, "Incomplete Recovery and Individualized Responses of the Human Distal Gut Microbiota to Repeated Antibiotic Perturbation," *Proceedings of the National Academy of Sciences* 108 (March 2011, Suppl 1): 4554–61.

12. M. Sharland, SACAR Pediatric Subgroup, "The Use of Antibacterials in Children: A Report of the Specialist Advisory Committee on Antimicrobial Resistance (SACAR) Paediatric Subgroup," *Journal of Antimicrobial Chemotherapy* 60 (August 2007, Suppl 1): i15–26; L. F. McCaig, R. E. Besser, J. M. Hughes, et al., "Trends in Antimicrobial Prescribing Rates for Children and Adolescents," *Journal of the American Medical Association* 287, no. 23 (June 19, 2002): 3096–102; J. Penders, C. Thijs, C. Vink, et al., "Factors Influencing the Composition of the Intestinal Microbiota in Early Infancy," *Pediatrics* 118, no. 2 (August 2006): 511–21.

13. L. Trasande, J. Blustein, M. Liu, et al., "Infant Antibiotic Exposures and

Early-Life Body Mass," *International Journal of Obesity* 37, no. 1 (January 2013): 16–23.

14. A. L. Hersh, D. J. Shapiro, A. T. Pavia, et al., "Antibiotic Prescribing in Ambulatory Pediatrics in the United States," *Pediatrics* 128, no. 6 (December 2011): 1053–61; M. L. Barnett and J. A. Linder, "Antibiotic Prescribing to Adults with Sore Throat in the United States, 1997–2010," *Journal of the American Medical Association Internal Medicine* 174, no. 1 (Jan. 2014):138–40; A. C. Nyquist, R. Gonzales, J. F. Steiner, et al., "Antibiotic Prescribing for Children with Colds, Upper Respiratory Tract Infections, and Bronchitis," *Journal of the American Medical Association* 279, no. 11 (March 1998): 875–77.

15. C. Jernberg, S. Lofmark, C. Edlund, et al., "Long-Term Impacts of Antibiotic Exposure on the Human Intestinal Microbiota," *Microbiology* 156, pt. 11 (November 2010): 3216–23; Dethlefsen, et al., "The Pervasive Effects of an Antibiotic," e280; Dethlefsen and Relman, "Incomplete Recovery," 4554–61.

16. H. E. Jakobsson, C. Jernberg, A. F. Andersson, et al., "Short-Term Antibiotic Treatment Has Differing Long-Term Impacts on the Human Throat and Gut Microbiome," *Public Library of Science One* 5, no. 3 (March 2010): e9836; M. Blaser, "Antibiotic Overuse: Stop the Killing of Beneficial Bacteria," *Nature* 476 (August 2011): 393–94; C. Jernberg, S. Lofmark, C. Edlund, et al., "Long-Term Ecological Impacts of Antibiotic Administration on the Human Intestinal Microbiota," *International Society for Microbial Ecology Journal* 1, no. 1 (May 2007): 56–66.

17. G. Ternak, "Antibiotics May Act as Growth/Obesity Promoters in Humans as an Inadvertent Result of Antibiotic Pollution?" *Medical Hypotheses* 64, no. 1 (2005): 14–16; M. J. Blaser and S. Falkow, "What Are the Consequences of the Disappearing Human Microbiota?" *National Review of Microbiology* 7, no. 12 (December 2009): 887–94; T. Jukes, "Antibiotics in Animal Feeds and Animal Production," *Bioscience* 22 (1972): 526–34.

18. Blaser, "What Are the Consequences?"

19. I Cho, S. Yamanishi, L Cox, et al., "Antibiotics in Early Life Alter the Murine Colonic Microbiome and Adiposity," *Nature* 488 (August 2012): 621–26; Y. Nobel, L. Cox, I. Tietler, et al., "Early-Life Pulsed Antibiotic Treatment as a Contributor to Enhanced Weight Gain and Bone Growth in Mice," Oral abstract session: Bacterial Pathogenesis and Virulence, IDSA Annual Meeting, Boston, 2011.

20. H. R. Gaskins, C. T. Collier, and D. B. Anderson, "Antibiotics As Growth Promotants: Mode of Action," *Animal Biotechnology* 13, no. 1 (May 2002): 29–42.

21. R. Laxminarayan, A. Duse, C. Wattal, et al., "Antibiotic Resistance—The Need for Global Solutions," *Lancet Infectious Diseases* 13, no. 12 (December 2013): 1057–98.

22. S. J. Howard, M. Catchpole, J. Watson, et al., "Antibiotic Resistance: Global Response Needed," *Lancet Infectious Diseases* 13, no. 12 (2013): 1001–1003.

23. Laxminarayan, et al., "Antibiotic Resistance," 1065.

24. Accessed December 10, 2014, www.fda.gov/drugs/resourcesforyou/consumers/ucm143568.htm. U.S. Department of Health and Human Services, Centers for Disease Control and Prevention, "Antibiotic Resistance Threats in the United States, 2013," accessed December 10, 2014, www.cdc.gov/drugresistance/threat-report-2013/pdf/ar-threats-2013-508.pdf.

25. K. M. Shea, "Antibiotic Resistance: What Is the Impact of Agricultural Uses of Antibiotics on Children's Health?" *Pediatrics* 112, 1 pt. 2 (July 2003): 253–58; Laxminarayan, et al., "Antibiotic Resistance," 1057–98.

26. A. R. Nisha, "Antibiotic Residues: A Global Health Hazard," *Veterinary World* 1, no. 12 (2008): 375–77; X. Ye, H. S. Weinburg, and M. T. Meyer, "Trace Analysis of Trimethoprim and Sulfonamide, Macrolide, Quinolone, and Tetracycline Antibiotics in Chlorinated Drinking Water Using Liquid Chromatography Electrospray Tandem Mass Spectrometry," *Anayticl Chemistry* 79, no. 3 (February 2007): 1135–44; P. L. Ruegg, "Antimicrobial Residues and Resistance: Understanding and Managing Drug Usage on Dairy Farms," University of Wisconsin, Dept. of Dairy Science, accessed December 9, 2013, milkquality.wisc.edu/wp-content/uploads/2011/09/Antimicrobial-Residues-and-Resistance-2013.pdf.

27. M. T. Bailey and C. L. Coe, "Maternal Separation Disrupts the Integrity of the Intestinal Microflora in Infant Rhesus Monkeys," *Developmental Psychobiology* 35, no. 2 (September 1999): 146–55; M. T. Bailey, G. R. Lubach, and C. L. Coe, "Prenatal Stress Alters Bacterial Colonization of the Gut in Infant Monkeys," *Journal of Pediatric Gastroenterology and Nutrition* 38, no. 4 (April 2004): 414–21; W. E. Moore, E. P. Cato, and L. V. Holdeman, "Some Current Concepts in Intestinal Bacteriology," *American Journal of Clinical Nutrition* 31 (October 1978, 10 Suppl): S33–42; M. T. Bailey, S. E. Dowd, J. D. Galley, et al., "Exposure to a Social Stressor Alters the Structure of the Intestinal Microbiota: Implications for Stressor-Induced Immunomodulation," *Brain, Behavior, and Immunity* 25, no. 3 (March 2011): 397–407; N. N. Lizko, "Stress and Intestinal Microflora." *Nahrung* 31, nos. 5–6 (1987): 443–47.

28. H. Eutamene and L. Bueno, "Role of Probiotics in Correcting Abnormalities of Colonic Flora Induced by Stress," *Gut* 56, no. 11 (November 2007): 1495–97; A. C. Logan and M. Katzman, "Major Depressive Disorder: Probiotics May Be an Adjuvant Therapy," *Medical Hypotheses* 64, no. 3 (2005): 533–38; J. D. Soderholm and M. H. Perdue, "Stress and Gastrointestinal Tract. II. Stress and Intestinal Barrier Function," *American Journal of Physiology Gastrointestinal and Liver Physiology* 280, no. 1 (January 2001): G7–G13.

29. M. Zareie, K. Johnson-Henry, J. Jury, et al., "Probiotics Prevent Bacterial Translocation and Improve Intestinal Barrier Function in Rats Following Chronic Psychological Stress," *Gut* 55, no. 11 (November 2006):1553–60.

30. A. Ait-Belgnaoui, H. Durand, C. Cartier, et al., "Prevention of Gut Leakiness by a Probiotic Treatment Leads to Attenuated HPA Response to an Acute Psy-

chological Stress in Rats," *Psychoneuroendocrinology* 37, no. 11 (November 2012): 1885–95.

31. T. Mitsuoka, "Intestinal Flora and Human Health," *Asia Pacific Journal of Clinical Nutrition* 15, no. 1 (1996): 2–9; E. J. Woodmansey, "Intestinal Bacteria and Ageing." *Journal of Applied Microbiolology* 102, no. 5 (May 2007): 1178–86; T. Mitsuoka, "Bifidobacteria and Their Role in Human Health," *Journal of Industrial Microbiology*, no. 6 (1990): 263–68.

32. F. He, A. C. Ouwehand, E. Isolauri, et al., "Differences in Composition and Mucosal Adhesion of Bifidobacteria Isolated from Healthy Adults and Healthy Seniors," *Current Microbiology* 43, no. 5 (November 2001): 351–54.

33. M. Aseeri, T. Schroeder, J. Kramer, et al., "Gastric Acid Suppression by Proton Pump Inhibitors as a Risk Factor for *Clostridium difficile*-Associated Diarrhea in Hospitalized Patients," *American Journal of Gastroenterology* 103, no. 9 (September 2008): 2308–13; S. Dial, J. A. Delaney, V. Schnieder, et al., "Proton Pump Inhibitor Use and Risk of Community-Acquired *Clostridium difficile*-Associated Disease Defined by Prescription for Oral Vancomycin Therapy," *Canadian Medical Association Journal* 175, no. 7 (September 2006):745–48, accessed December 17, 2013, http://www.mayoclinic.com/health/c-difficile/DS00736.

34. R. J. Valuck and J. M. Ruscin, "A Case-Control Study on Adverse Effects: H2 Blocker or Proton Pump Inhibitor Use and Risk of Vitamin B12 Deficiency in Older Adults," *Journal of Clinical Epidemiology* 57, no. 4 (April 2004): 422–28.

35. K. W. Altman, V. Chhaya, N. D. Hamme, et al., "Effect of Proton Pump Inhibitor Pantoprazole on Growth and Morphology of Oral Lactobacillus Strains," *Laryngoscope* 118, no. 4 (April 2008): 599–604.

36. W. K. Lo and W. W. Chan, "Proton Pump Inhibitor Use and the Risk of Small Intestinal Bacterial Overgrowth: A Meta-Analysis," *Clinical Gastroenterology and Hepatology* 11, no. 5 (May 2013): 483–90.

37. Accessed December 18, 2013, http://www.ewg.org/research/body-burden-pollution-newborns.

38. S. O. Duke and S. B. Powles, "Glyphosate: A Once-in-a-Century Herbicide," *Pest Management Science* 64, no. 4 (April 2008): 319–25.

39. A. Samsel and S. Seneff, "Glyphosate's Suppression of Cytochrome P450 Enzymes and Amino Acid Biosynthesis by the Gut Microbiome Pathways to Modern Diseases," *Entropy* 15 (2013): 1416–63; A. A. Shehata, W. Schrodl, A. A. Aldin, et al., "The Effect of Glyphosate on Potential Pathogens and Beneficial Members of Poultry Microbiota in Vitro," *Current Microbiology* 66, no. 4 (April 2013): 350–58.

40. A. O. Summers, J. Wireman, M. J. Vimy, et al., "Mercury Released from Dental 'Silver' Fillings Provokes an Increase in Mercury- and Antibiotic-Resistant Bacteria in Oral and Intestinal Floras of Primates," *Antimicrobial Agents and Chemotherapy* 37, no. 4 (April 1993): 825–34.

41. M. B. Abou-Donia, E. M. El-Masry, A. A. Abdel-Rahman, et al., "Splenda

Alters Gut Microflora and Increases Intestinal p-Glycoprotein and Cytochrome p-450 in Male Rats," *Journal of Toxicological Environmental Health Part A* 71, no. 21 (2008): 1415–29.

42. M. Arciello, M. Gori, R. Maggio, et al., "Environmental Pollution: A Tangible Risk for NAFLD Pathogenesis," *International Journal of Molecular Science* 14, no. 11 (November 2013): 22052–66.

43. Environmental Working Group, "Current Science on Public Exposures to Toxic Chemicals," testimony of Kenneth A. Cook, accessed February 5, 2014, http://www.epw.senate.gov/public/index.cfm?FuseAction=Files.View&FileStore_id=31bcb6cf-26ff-4415-b04d-87988118af33.

Chapter 4: The Proper Care and Feeding of Your Own Gut Bacteria

1. P. D. Cani, "Selective Increases of Bifidobacteria in Gut Microflora Improve High-Fat-Diet-Induced Diabetes in Mice through a Mechanism Associated with Endotoxaemia," *Diabetologia* 50, no. 11 (November 2007): 2374–83; M. Kalliomaki, M. C. Collado, S. Salminen, et al., "Early Differences in Fecal Microbiota Composition in Children May Predict Overweight," *American Journal of Clinical Nutrition* 87, no. 3 (March 2008): 534–38; X. Wu, C. Ma, L. Han, et al., "Molecular Characterisation of the Faecal Microbiota in Patients with Type II Diabetes," *Current Microbiology* 61, no. 1 (July 2010): 69–78.

2. Y. Kadooka, M. Sato, K. Imaizumi, et al., "Regulation of Abdominal Adiposity by Probiotics (*Lactobacillus gasseri* SBT2055) in Adults with Obese Tendencies in a Randomized Controlled Trial," *European Journal of Clinical Nutrition* 64, no. 6 (June 2010): 636–43.

3. R. Luoto, M. Kalliomaki, K. Laitinen, et al., "The Impact of Perinatal Probiotic Intervention on the Development of Overweight and Obesity: Follow-up Study from Birth to 10 Years." *International Journal of Obesity* 34, no. 10 (October 2010): 1531–37.

4. K. Laitinen, T. Poussa, E. Isolauri, et al., "Probiotics and Dietary Counselling Contribute to Glucose Regulation during and after Pregnancy: A Randomised Controlled Trial," *British Journal of Nutrition* 101, no. 11 (June 2009): 1679–87.

5. N. P. McNulty, T. Yatsunenko, A. Hsiao, et al., "The Impact of a Consortium of Fermented Milk Strains on the Gut Microbiome of Gnotobiotic Mice and Monozygotic Twins," *Science Translational Medicine* 3, no. 106 (October 2011): 106ra106.

6. M. Roberfroid, G. R. Gibson, L. Hoyles, et al., "Prebiotic Effects: Metabolic and Health Benefits," *British Journal of Nutrition* 104 (August 2010, Suppl.2): S1–63.

7. P. D. Cani, E. Joly, Y. Horsmans, et al., "Oligofructose Promotes Satiety in Healthy Human: A Pilot Study," *European Journal of Clinical Nutrition* 60, no. 5 (May 2006): 567–72.

8. P. D. Cani, E. Lecourt, E. M. Dewulf, et al., "Gut Microbiota Fermentation of Prebiotics Increases Satietogenic and Incretin Gut Peptide Production with

Consequences for Appetite Sensation and Glucose Response after a Meal," *American Journal of Clinical Nutrition* 90, no. 5 (November 2009): 1236–43.

Chapter 5: Your Gut Connection to Obesity and Other Common Conditions

1. J. B. Furness, W. E. Kunze, and N. Clerc, "Nutrient Tasting and Signaling Mechanisms in the Gut. II. The Intestine As a Sensory Organ: Neural, Endocrine, and Immune Responses," *American Journal of Physiology* 277, no. 5, pt.1 (November 1999): G922–28.

2. G. S. Hotamisiliqil, "Inflammation and Metabolic Disorders," *Nature* 444 (December 2006): 860–67.

3. Accessed December, 19, 2013: http://www.uptodate.com/contents/constipation -in-adults-beyond-the-basics.

4. C. Chassard, M. Dapigny, K. P. Scott, et al., "Functional Dysbiosis within the Gut Microbiota of Patients with Constipated-Irritable Bowel Syndrome," *Alimentary Pharmacology and Therapeutics* 35, no. 7 (April 2012): 828–38.

5. Accessed December 19, 2013: http://digestive.niddk.nih.gov/ddiseases/pubs/ibs/.

6. S. Dial, J. A. Delaney, V. Schneider, et al., "Proton Pump Inhibitor Use and Risk of Community-Acquired *Clostridium difficile*–Associated Disease Defined by Prescription for Oral Vancomycin Therapy," *Canadian Medical Association Journal.* 175, no. 7 (September 2006): 745–48.

7. A. Chocarro Martinez, F. Galindo Tobal, G. Ruiz-Irastorza, et al., "Risk Factors for Esophageal Candidiasis," *European Journal of Clinical Microbiology and Infectious Diseases* 19, no. 2 (February 2000): 96–100.

8. L. E. Tarqownik, L. M. Lix, C. J. Metqe, et al., "Use of Proton Pump Inhibitors and Risk of Osteoporosis-Related Fractures." *Canadian Medical Association Journal* 179, no. 4 (August 2008): 319–26.

9. S. E. Gulmez, A. Holm, H. Frederiksen, et al., "Use of Proton Pump Inhibitors and the Risk of Community-Acquired Pneumonia: A Population-Based Case-Control Study," *Archives of Internal Medicine* 167, no. 9 (May 2007): 950–55.

10. R. J. Valuck and J. M. Ruscin, "A Case-Control Study on Adverse Effects: H2 Blocker or Proton Pump Inhibitor Use and Risk of Vitamin B12 Deficiency in Older Adults," *Journal of Clinical Epidemiology* 57, no. 4 (April 2004): 422–28.

Chapter 6: The Gut-Brain Connection

1. J. F. Cryan and T. G. Dinan, "Mind-Altering Microorganisms: The Impact of the Gut Microbiota on Brain and Behaviour," *National Review of Neuroscience* 13, no. 10 (October 2012): 701–12.

2. M. Maes, M. Berk, L. Goehler, et al., "Depression and Sickness Behavior Are Janus-Faced Responses to Shared Inflammatory Pathways," *Bio Med Central Medicine* 10 (June 2012): 66; P. Bercik, E. F. Verdu, J. A. Foster, et al., "Chronic Gastrointestinal Inflammation Induces Anxiety-like Behavior and Alters Central Nervous System Biochemistry in Mice," *Gastroenterology* 139, no. 6 (December 2010): 2102–12.e1.

3. A. C. Logan and M. Katzman, "Major Depressive Disorder: Probiotics May Be an Adjuvant Therapy," *Medical Hypotheses* 64, no. 3 (2005): 533–38; A. V. Rao, A. C. Bested, T. M. Beaulne, et al., "A Randomized, Double-blind, Placebo-controlled Pilot Study of a Probiotic in Emotional Symptoms of Chronic Fatigue Syndrome," *Gut Pathogens* 19, no. 1 (March 2009): 6; M. Messaoudi, R. Lalonde, N. Violle, et al., "Assessment of Psychotropic-like Properties of a Probiotic Formulation (Lactobacillus helveticus R0052 and Bifidobacterium longum R0175) in Rats and Human Subjects," *British Journal of Nutrition* 105, no. 5 (March 2011): 755–64.

4. Logan and Katzman, "Major Depressive Disorder."

5. T. G. Dinan, C. Stanton, and J. F. Cryan, "Psychobiotics: A Novel Class of Psychotropic," *Biological Psychiatry* 74, no. 10 (November 2013): 720–26.

6. M. Lyte, "Probiotics Function Mechanistically as Delivery Vehicles for Neuroactive Compounds: Microbial Endocrinology in the Design and Use of Probiotics," *Bioessays* 33, no. 8 (August 2011): 574–81; A. Schousboe and H. S. Waagepetersen, "GABA: Homeostatic and Pharmacological Aspects," *Progressive Brain Research* 160 (2007): 9–19; V. V. Roshchina, "Evolutionary Considerations of Neurotransmitters in Microbial, Plant, and Animal Cells," *Microbial Endocrinology: Interkingdom Signaling in Infectious Disease and Health,* ed. Lyte M, Freestone PPE (New York: Springer, 17–52).

7. L. Desbonnet, L. Garret, G. Clarke, et al., "The probiotic *Bifidobacteria infantis*: An assessment of potential antidepressant properties in the rat," *Journal of Psychiatric Research* 43, no. 2 (December 2008): 164–74.

8. L. Desbonnet, L. Garret, G. Clarke, et al., "Effects of the Probiotic *Bifidobacterium infantis* in the Maternal Separation Model of Depression," *Neuroscience* 170, no. 4 (November 2010): 1179–88; J. A. Bravo, P. Forsythe, M. V. Chew, et al., "Ingestion of Lactobacillus Strain Regulates Emotional Behavior and Central GABA Receptor Expression in a Mouse via the Vagus Nerve," *Proceedings of the National Academy of Sciences of the United States* 108, no. 38 (September 2011): 16050–55.

9. P. Bercik, E. Denou, J. Collins, et al., "The Intestinal Microbiota Affect Central Levels of Brain-derived Neurotropic Factor and Behavior in Mice," *Gastroenterology* 141, no. 2 (August 2011): 599–609, 609.e1–3.

10. N. Sudo, Y. Chida, Y. Aiba, et al., "Postnatal Microbial Colonization Programs the Hypothalamic-Pituitary-Adrenal System for Stress Response in Mice." *Journal of Physiology* 558, pt. 1 (July 2004): 263–75.

11. Dinan et al., "Psychobiotics."

12. Messaoudi, et al., "Assessment of Psychotropic-like Properties," D. Benton, C. Williams, and A. Brown, "Impact of Consuming a Milk Drink Containing a Probiotic on Mood and Cognition," *European Journal of Clinical Nutrition* 61, no. 3 (March 2007): 355–61; Rao et al., "A Randomized, Double-blind."

13. K. Tillisch, J. Labus, L. Kilpatrick, et al., "Consumption of Fermented Milk Product with Probiotic Modulates Brain Activity." *Gastroenterology* 144, no. 7 (June 2013): 1394–401, 1401.e1–4.

14. K. J. Davey, S. M. O'Mahoney, H. Schellekens, et al., "Gender-dependent Consequences of Chronic Olanzapine in the Rat: Effects on Body Weight, Inflammatory, Metabolic and Microbiota Parameters," *Psychopharmacology* 221, no. 1 (May 2012): 155–69.

Chapter 7: The Skinny on Food

1. J. A. Hawrelak and S. P. Myers, "The Causes of Intestinal Dysbiosis: A Review," *Alternative Medicine Review* 9, no. 2 (June 2004): 180–97; C. Erridge, T. Attina, C.M. Spickett, et al., "A High-Fat Meal Induces Low-Grade Endotoxemia: Evidence of a Novel Mechanism of Postprandial Inflammation," *American Journal of Clinical Nutrition* 86, no. 5 (November 2007): 1286–92.
2. P. J. Turnbaugh, V. K. Ridaura, J. J. Faith, et al., "The Effect of Diet on the Human Gut Microbiome: A Metagenomic Analysis in Humanized Gnotobiotic Mice," *Science Translational Medicine* 1, no. 6 (November 2009): 6ra14.
3. A. P. Simopoulos, "Omega-3 Fatty Acids in Health and Disease and in Growth and Development," *American Journal of Clinical Nutrition* 54, no. 3 (September 1991): 438–63.
4. Ibid.
5. D. S. Weigle , P. A. Breen, C. C. Matthys, et al., "A High-Protein Diet Induces Sustained Reductions in Appetite, ad libitum Caloric Intake, and Body Weight Despite Compensatory Changes in Diurnal Plasma Leptin and Ghrelin Concentrations," *American Journal of Clinical Nutrition* 82, no. 1 (July 2005): 41–48.

Chapter 11: Skinny Gut Supplements

1. G. Danaei, E. L. Ding, D. Mozaffarian, et al., "The Preventable Causes of Death in the United States: Comparative Risk Assessment of Dietary, Lifestyle, and Metabolic Risk Factors," *Public Library of Sciences Medicine* 6, no. 4 (April 2009): e1000058.
2. C. Chapman, G. R. Gibson, I. Rowland, et al., "Health Benefits of Probiotics: Are Mixtures More Effective than Single Strains?" *European Journal of Nutrition* 50, no. 1 (February 2011): 1–17.

Appendix: Gut Science with Dr. Smith

1. V. K. Ridaura, J. J. Faith, F. F. Rey, et al., "Gut Microbiota from Twins Discordant for Obesity Modulate Metabolism in Mice," *Science* 341 (September 2013): 1241214.
2. M. J. Keenan, J. Zhou, K. L. McCutcheon, et al., "Effects of Resistant Starch, a Non-Digestible Fermentable Fiber, on Reducing Body Fat," *Obesity* 14, no. 9 (September 2006): 1523–34.
3. E. Le Chatelier, T. Nielsen, J. Qin, et al., "Richness of Human Gut Microbiome Correlates with Metabolic Markers," *Nature* 500 (August 2013): 541–46.
4. Ibid., p. 544.
5. C. Manichanh, L. Rigottier-Gois, E. Bonnaud, et al., "Reduced Diversity of

Faecal Microbiota in Crohn's Disease Revealed by a Metagenomic Approach," *Gut* 55, no. 2 (February 2006): 205–11; P. Lepage, R. Hasler, M. E. Spehlmann, et al., "Twin Study Indicates Loss of Interaction between Microbiota and Mucosa of Patients with Ulcerative Colitis," *Gastroenterology* 141, no. 1 (July 2011): 227–36; M. J. Claesson, I. B. Jeffrey, S. Conde, et al., "Gut Microbiota Composition Correlates with Diet and Health in the Elderly," *Nature* 488 (August 2012): 178–84; P. J. Turnbaugh, M. Hamady, T. Yatsuneko, et al., "A Core Gut Microbiome in Obese and Lean Twins," *Nature* 457 (January 2009): 480–84; I. Cho, S. Yamanishi, I. Cox, et al., "Antibiotics in Early Life Alter the Murine Colonic Microbiome and Adiposity," *Nature* 488 (August 2012): 621–26; T. A. Ajslev, C. S. Andersen, M. Gamborg, et al., "Childhood Overweight after Establishment of the Gut Microbiota: The Role of Delivery Mode, Pre-pregnancy Weight and Early Administration of Antibiotics," *International Journal of Obesity* 35, no. 4 (April 2011): 522–29.

6. N. Fei and L. Zhao, "An Opportunistic Pathogen Isolated from the Gut of an Obese Human Causes Obesity in Germfree Mice," *International Society for Microbial Ecology Journal* 7, no. 4 (April 2013): 880–84.

7. P. D. Cani, R. Bibiloni, C. Knauf, et al., "Changes in Gut Microbiota Control Metabolic Endotoxemia-Induced Inflammation in High-fat Diet-Induced Obesity and Diabetes in Mice," *Diabetes* 57, no. 6 (June 2008): 1470–81; P. D. Cani, J. Amar, M. A. Iglesias, et al., "Metabolic Endotoxemia Initiates Obesity and Insulin Resistance," *Diabetes* 57, no. 7 (July 2007): 1761–72.

8. Cani, et al., "Changes in Gut Microbiota."

9. O. S. Al-Attas, N. M. Al-Daghri, K. Al_rubeaan, et al., "Changes in Endotoxin Levels in T2DM Subjects on Anti-Diabetic Therapies," *Cardiovascular Diabetology* 8 (April 2009): 20; A. Gummesson, L. M. Calrsson, L. H. Storlien, et al., "Intestinal Permeability Is Associated with Visceral Adiposity in Healthy Women," *Obesity* 19, no. 11 (November 2011): 2280–82.

10. J. Amar, M. Serino, C. Lange, et al., "Involvement of Tissue Bacteria in the Onset of Diabetes in Humans: Evidence for a Concept," *Diabetologia* 54, no. 12 (December 2011): 3055–61.

11. A. Vrieze, E. Van Nood, F. Holleman, et al., "Transfer of Intestinal Microbiota from Lean Donors Increases Insulin Sensitivity in Individuals with Metabolic Syndrome," *Gastroenterology* 143, no. 4 (October 2012): 913–16.e7.

12. H. V. Lin, A. Frassetto, E. J. Kowalik Jr., et al., "Butyrate and Propionate Protect Against Diet-induced Obesity and Regulate Gut Hormones via Free Fatty Acid Receptor 3–Independent Mechanisms," *Public Library of Sciences One* 7, no. 4 (2012): e35240.

13. K. M. Maslowski and C. R. MacKay, "Diet, Gut Microbiota and Immune Responses," *Natural Immunology* 12, no. 1 (January 2011): 5–9.

14. Ibid.

15. J. King, Z. Zhang, M. W. Musch, et al., "Novel Role of the Vitamin D Receptor in Maintaining the Integrity of the Intestinal Mucosal Barrier," *American Jour-*

nal of Physiology Gastrointestinal and Liver Physiology 294, no. 1 (January 2008): G208–16.

16. W. Liu, Y. Chen, M. A. Golan, et al., "Intestinal Epithelial Vitamin D Receptor Signaling Inhibits Experimental Colitis," *Journal of Clinical Investigation* 123, no. 9 (September 2013): 3983–96.

INDEX

ABOUT THE AUTHORS

BRENDA WATSON, C.N.C., has dedicated her career for more than twenty years to helping people achieve vibrant, lasting health through improved digestive function. A dynamic health advocate and celebrated public television health educator, she is among the foremost authorities in America on optimum nutrition, digestion, and natural detoxification methods. She is the author of *The Fiber35 Diet*, a *New York Times* bestseller, and eight other books on gut-related health.

LEONARD SMITH, M.D., is a board-certified, general, gastrointestinal, and vascular surgeon. Currently, Dr. Smith is on the volunteer faculty at the University of Miami Department of Surgery and Department of Integrative Medicine.

JAMEY JONES is a health and science writer with a background in botany and nutrition. She is the coauthor of *Heart of Perfect Health*, *The Road to Perfect Health*, and *Gut Solutions*, second edition, all with Brenda Watson.